THE PEACEFUL BRAIN ART BOOK

Dedication

To my family, for always believing in me. To my best friends, who accept me and love me with all my flaws. To my love – thank you for your encouragement, your patience and your support. And to my mum – your love has carried me more than you'll ever know.

First published in Great Britain in 2026 by Ilex,
an imprint of Octopus Publishing Group Ltd
Carmelite House
50 Victoria Embankment
London EC4Y 0DZ
www.octopusbooks.co.uk

An Hachette UK Company
www.hachette.co.uk

The authorized representative in the EEA is Hachette Ireland, 8 Castlecourt Centre, Dublin 15, D15 XTP3, Ireland (email: info@hbgi.ie)

Distributed in the US by Hachette Book Group, 1290 Avenue of the Americas, 4th and 5th Floors, New York, NY 10104

Distributed in Canada by Canadian Manda Group, 664 Annette St, Toronto, Ontario, Canada M6S 2C8

ISBN: 978-1-84601-742-1
eISBN: 978-1-84601-762-9

A CIP catalogue record for this book is available from the British Library.

Printed and bound in China.

10 9 8 7 6 5 4 3 2 1

Commissioning Editor: Emma Hanson
Senior Editor: Leanne Bryan
Art Director: Ben Gardiner
Copyeditor: Emma Clegg
Designer: JC Lanaway
Photographer: Elijah Edwards
Photo Producer: Mark Albini
Production Manager: Caroline Alberti

MIX
Paper | Supporting responsible forestry
FSC www.fsc.org FSC® C008047

Disclaimer

All reasonable care has been taken in the preparation of this book, but the information it contains is not intended to take the place of treatment by a qualified medical practitioner.

Before making any changes in your health regime, always consult a doctor. While all the therapies detailed in this book are completely safe if done correctly, you must seek professional advice if you are in any doubt about any medical condition. Any application of the ideas and information contained in this book is at the reader's sole discretion and risk.

Demi Dawkins

THE PEACEFUL BRAIN ART BOOK

55 self-soothing art exercises for ADHD, autism and anxiety

ilex

Contents

Introduction 7
Why art helps create a peaceful brain 8
How to create a peaceful practice 10

Grounding & Calm 15
Introduction 16
1. Emotional flow lines 18
2. Breath & brush 20
3. Weighted colour wash 22
4. Circles of safety 24
5. Tracing hands 26
6. Bilateral drawing 28
7. Colour breathing 30
8. Soothing symmetry 32
9. Scribble release 34
10. Paint with texture 36

Releasing Anxiety 39
Introduction 40
11. Storm to stillness 42
12. Anxiety box 44
13. Tear & transform 46
14. Knot & untangle 48
15. Colour-mapping feelings 50
16. Wave motion drawing 52
17. Mindful mandalas 54
18. Shatter & repair 56
19. Mindful dots 58
20. Puddles of imperfection 60

Embracing Uncertainty 63
Introduction 64
21. Blindfold art 66
22. Swap hands drawing 68
23. The pebble exercise 70
24. Chance colours 72
25. Ink bloom experiment 74
26. Follow the music 76
27. Surface & surrender 78
28. Spill & respond 80
29. Chaos to composition 82
30. The pebble mandala 84

Neurodivergent Strengths 87
Introduction 88
31. Trace the overwhelm 90
32. The quiet space 92
33. Strength self-portrait 94
34. Sensory collage 96
35. Feeling to flow 98
36. Hyperfocus drawing 100
37. Routine mandala 102
38. Hidden message layer 104
39. Touch & trace 106
40. Sound shapes 108
41. Three-tool challenge 110
42. Pixel pieces 112
43. Stained-glass emotions 114

Hope, Joy & Reflection 117
Introduction 118
44. Gratitude spiral 120
45. Future window 122
46. Joyful colour bursts 124
47. Light rays 126
48. Self-love doodles 128
49. Mindset collage 130
50. Calm landscape 132
51. Growth rings 134
52. Affirmation poster 136
53. Celebration confetti 138
54. Fruitful study 140
55. Flowers as feelings 142

Acknowledgements 144
Further reading 144

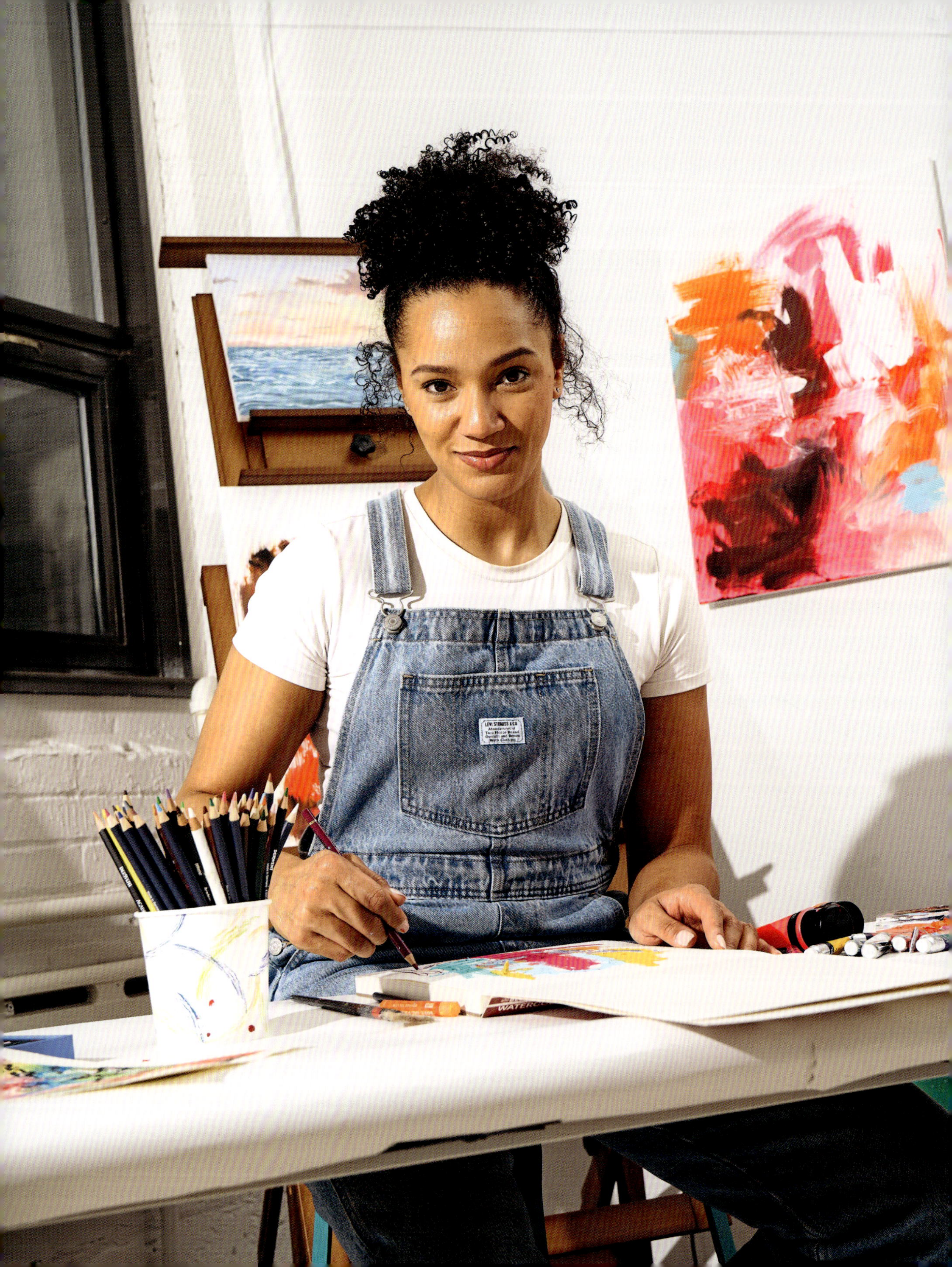

Introduction

For as long as I can remember, my mind has been a beautifully buzzing place – full of colour, emotion, curiosity and, at times, intensity. When I was later diagnosed with ADHD and autism, everything finally made sense. The overwhelm. The sensitivity. The craving for silence and space. But also the vivid imagination, the deep empathy, the intuition, and the hunger to express myself in ways words could never quite hold.

Art became my therapy long before I ever had the language to call it that.

When I paint or draw, something inside me settles. My brush becomes an extension of my inner world, translating feelings into flowing shapes and vibrant hues. Each piece becomes a breath, a prayer, a grounding ritual – a way to regulate, reflect and gently guide myself back into peace. Through pattern, texture and tone, I explore light, love, faith and the delicate balance between chaos and calm.

I created *The Peaceful Brain Art Book* to share the rituals and practices that have helped me feel anchored, especially on days when the world feels too loud or my mind moves too fast. These pages are filled with gentle creative exercises that mirror the same techniques I use to navigate overwhelm, release pressure and reconnect with myself.

Art has always been the tool that helps me give my hyperactivity, anxiety and emotions a safe place to land. Sometimes the simple act of colouring a shape or tracing a pattern is enough to steady my thoughts and ground my senses. This book was created with that intention: to offer you a safe, creative sanctuary you can return to whenever life begins to feel overwhelming.

Whether you're neurodivergent too, or simply sometimes overwhelmed by the noises and stresses of daily life, I hope this book becomes a place where you can slow down, breathe more deeply and remember that your mind – in all its depth and complexity – is a beautiful place to be.

Let us create peace – together.

With love and colour,

Demi x

Why art helps create a peaceful brain

Like therapy, art can be healing and grounding. It can provide language when words fall short. For me, art has become a way to express experiences or feelings that are too big, complex or intense for language alone.

As a marriage and family therapist in the mental health field, I've worked with people of many ages and backgrounds, especially in areas of relationships and trauma. Again and again I've seen how art can help people heal as it forges a path to a deeper connection and to emotional release and repair.

There is a scientific reason why this works. Art supports emotional processing and regulation and helps the brain release 'feel good' chemicals, lower stress levels, and learn new patterns of thinking and behaving.

How the brain works

To understand how art helps regulate emotions, it is helpful to understand how the brain works. Start by making a fist.

The front of your fist represents the **frontal lobe** – the part of the brain that helps you plan, make decisions and manage emotions.

Inside your fist is the **temporal lobe** and **hippocampus**, which organize memories.

Behind this lies the **parietal lobe**, which helps you understand physical sensations such as touch and pain.

The back of the fist is where the **occipital lobe** is found, responsible for vision and interpreting what we see.

Below this, at the base of the fist, is the **cerebellum**, responsible for movement and coordination, as well as learned patterns and habits.

All of these parts work together in one integrated system.

Within the brain lies a complex network of nerves called the limbic system, which controls emotional responses and your behaviour. Inside this system is a small, almond-shaped structure called the **amygdala**. This controls how you experience emotions like anxiety, anger and fear. It detects danger and controls our fight, flight or freeze responses.

The brain sends messages to the body through a highway called the spinal cord, which is connected to the brainstem. These messages are then passed to the autonomic nervous system, which has two branches:

- ⇛ The **sympathetic nervous system**, supporting activation and mobilization, known as 'fight or flight'.
- ⇛ The **parasympathetic nervous system**, supporting rest and recovery, known as 'rest and digest'.

Your brain can change

Your experiences, environment and daily routines can shape your brain. This is known as neuroplasticity. When you practise something new – like art, mindfulness or gratitude – you help your brain build new pathways. Over time this can help you respond differently to the same situations and even experience new emotions.

Why the body matters

The exercises in this book include body-based (somatic) approaches. This means paying attention to the sensations in the body and how these relate to your emotions. Somatic exercises include grounding, breathing exercises, gentle movement and mindfulness. As you work through the exercises, remember that they can have powerful positive impacts on your brain and emotions.

Art and the brain

Research shows that spending as little as 45 minutes creating art can lower stress hormones and help the body relax. New research shows that art can activate the brain's pleasure centres, while calming areas linked to threat and fear.

Being part of *The Peaceful Brain Art Book* is an honour that allows me to bring the benefits of art to an even wider audience.

Jovanna Penney

How to create a peaceful practice

A peaceful practice does not have to be perfect, aesthetic or consistent to be meaningful. It does not require hours of uninterrupted time, expensive materials or a dedicated studio space. What matters most is that it feels safe, grounding and supportive for you.

This book isn't about producing perfect artwork – it's about creating a space where your nervous system can settle, your mind can slow and your creativity can move without pressure. Your practice is not something to perform. It is something to return to.

Choosing your space

Start by choosing a place where you feel relatively comfortable. This could be a desk, a kitchen table, the floor, a corner of your bedroom or even your bed.

There is no 'correct' set-up – only what works for your body and mind on that day.

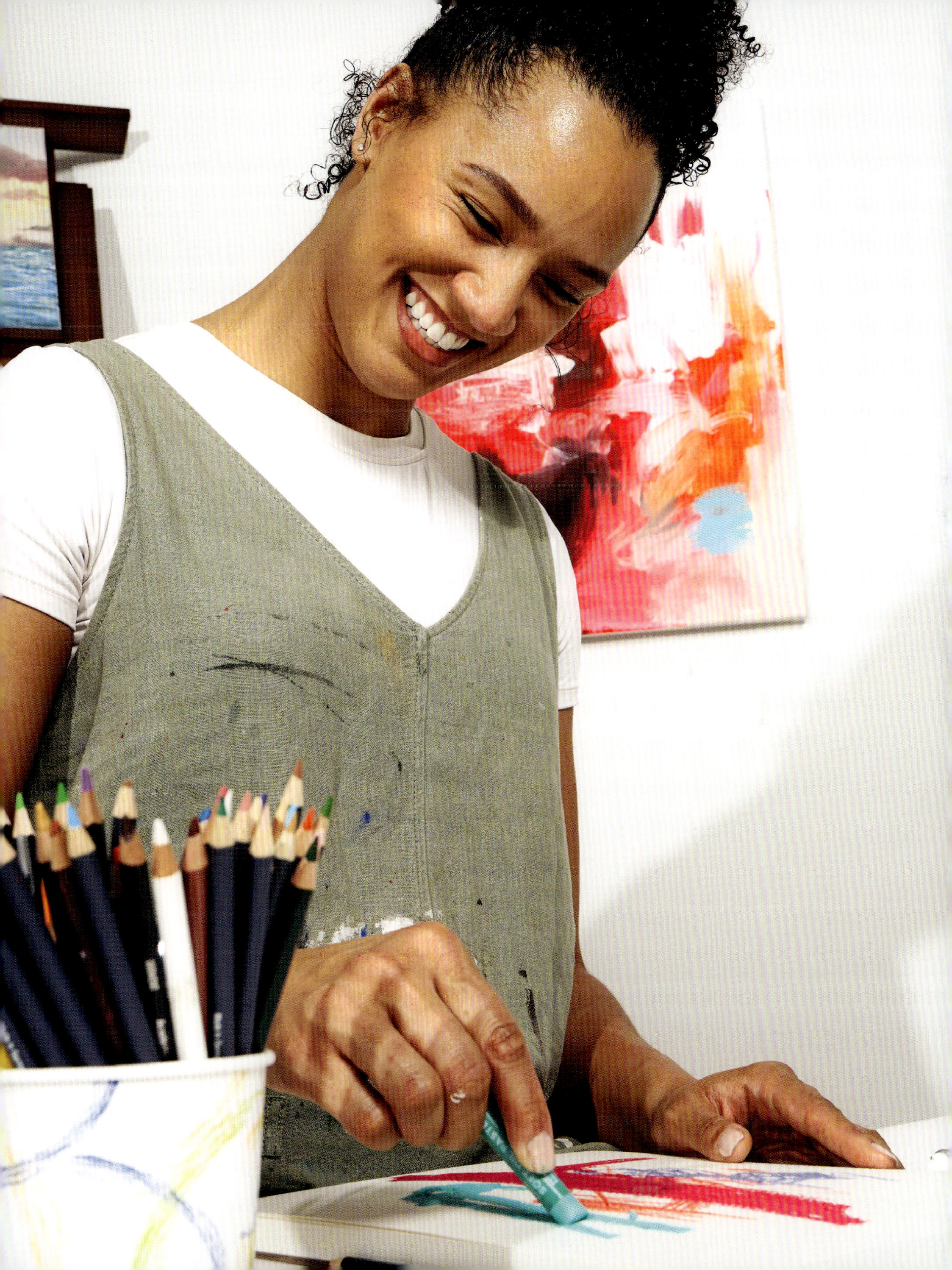

Creating a gentle beginning

Before you start any exercise, give yourself a moment to arrive.

This could be as simple as:

⇒ taking three slow breaths

⇒ placing your feet on the floor and noticing their contact

⇒ resting your hands on the paper before making a mark.

You don't need to feel calm before you begin. The practice is there to meet you where you are – busy mind, tired body, scattered thoughts and all.

Letting go of outcomes

One of the most important parts of a peaceful practice is letting go of the idea of a 'good' or 'successful' result.

These exercises are not tests – they are simply invitations.

If you notice judgement creeping in – whether it be about your skill, your speed or how the page looks – gently return your attention to your senses. Notice the movement of your hand, the sound of the pen or the feeling of the paper. Shifting from thinking to sensing is often where calm begins.

You are allowed to stop in the middle of an exercise. You are allowed to skip pages. You are allowed to return days later. Consistency does not mean doing it perfectly – it means coming back when you can.

Ending with care

When you finish, take a moment to pause before closing the book or putting your materials away. Notice how your body feels now, compared to when you started.

You might ask yourself:

⇛ Do I feel heavier, lighter, slower, steadier?

⇛ What changed, even slightly?

There is no need to analyse or interpret your work. Simply acknowledging the experience helps your nervous system register it as safe and complete.

A practice that grows with you

Your peaceful practice will change over time – just like you. Some days it may feel deeply calming. Other days it may simply feel neutral. Both are valid.

This book is not asking you to fix yourself or be more productive. It offers you a place to rest inside creativity, letting art be a companion instead of a demand.

Move gently. Go at your own pace. Let this practice belong to you.

CHAPTER 1

GROUNDING & CALM

Introduction

For many neurodivergent people, our minds can move quickly, jumping between thoughts, ideas, memories, sounds and sensations. While this can be a source of creativity, it can also lead to feelings of restlessness, overwhelm or disconnection from the body.

The exercises in this chapter are designed to help slow that internal pace and offer a sense of steadiness, returning you to the present moment, gently and without force.

Grounding means giving your nervous system something stable to rest on. Through simple, repetitive movements, sensory awareness, and intentional mark-making, the practices in this chapter invite your attention back into your hands, your breath, and the physical act of creating.

Some exercises may feel deeply soothing, while others help you feel more present. Calm can be subtle – it might show up as a softened jaw, a slower breath or a quieter inner dialogue. Small moments of calm accumulate over time.

Work slowly and take breaks when needed. There is no expectation to complete an exercise in one sitting, or to finish every page. Return to these practices whenever your body asks for rest, grounding or reassurance.

THERAPIST'S NOTE

Grounding is a mindful, self-soothing technique to encourage you to stay present and lessen the mental noise. Stress is stored in our bodies, yet as we rush around, we're not aware of the stress we are carrying. Grounding allows us to become aware of both the present moment as well as what is happening within our bodies. This is also called attunement – it helps us align with ourselves, guiding our thoughts, and supporting us in honouring and advocating for our own experiences. When our brains experience self-attunement or mindfulness, we lessen our cortisol stress response and release the 'feel good' neurotransmitters in our body.

This chapter invites you to explore different forms of mindfulness through the art exercises. These activities can help you step away from negative thoughts, practise acceptance instead of judgement, and develop more kindness and empathy towards yourself and others.

EXERCISE 1

Emotional flow lines

Slow, repetitive line movements can help the body feel calmer. They give the mind a simple, predictable rhythm to follow. This can ease overthinking and bring your attention back to what you are doing, through gentle movement.

INSTRUCTIONS

1. Choose three colours that match how you feel right now.
2. Paint long, overlapping strokes, or draw lines freely. Let them cross and weave.
3. Keep adding layers until the page begins to reflect your mood.
4. Add simple lines between the strokes to create rhythm and structure. You might add small circles, hatching or loose squiggles – choose what feels easy.

WHAT YOU NEED

⇒ Paper

⇒ Paints and brushes, pens, pencils or another material of choice

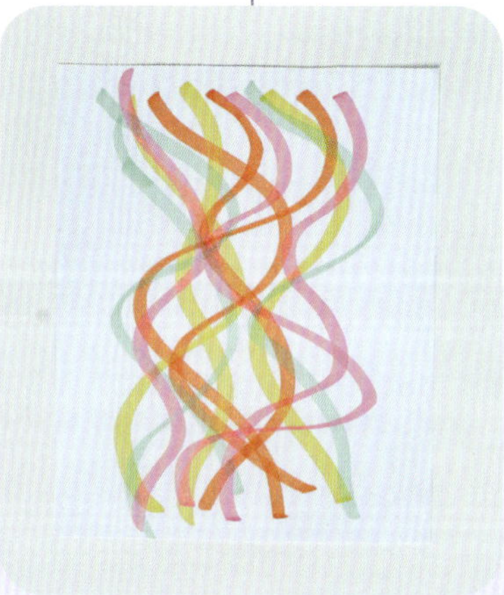

Alternative drawing

THERAPIST'S INSIGHT

When the brain completes this exercise, finishing the lines activates reward centres, helping you feel safe and satisfied, and releasing serotonin, the 'feel-good' hormone.

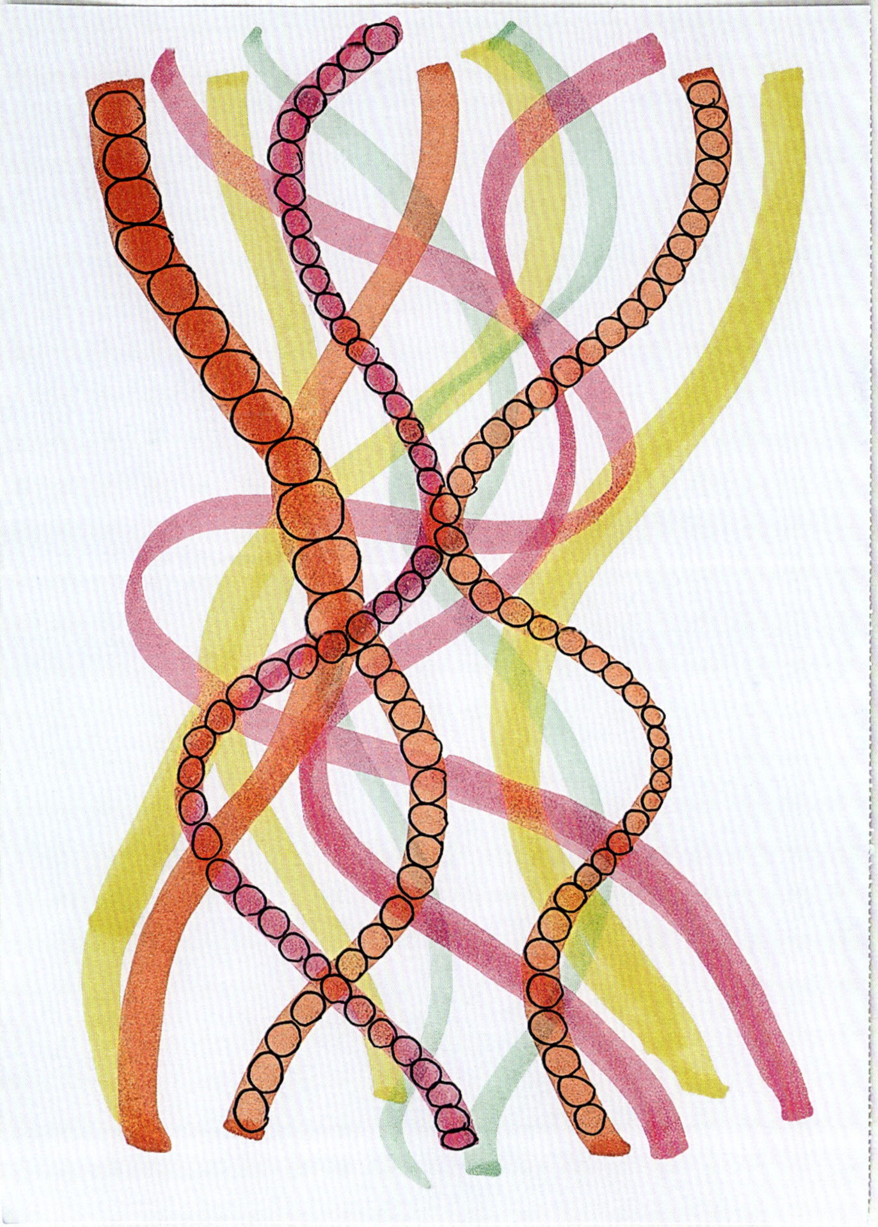

EXERCISE 2

Breath & brush

Moving the brush in time with your breathing can help your body feel calmer. It turns painting into a gentle, focused practice and can bring your attention back to your body when your mind feels overwhelmed.

INSTRUCTIONS

1. Dip your brush in paint, or choose a pen.
2. As you breathe in, move the brush upwards and outwards.
3. As you breathe out, move the brush downwards and inwards.
4. Continue painting or drawing in this breath-led rhythm.
5. Let the marks remain simple and unforced.

WHAT YOU NEED

⇒ Paper

⇒ Paint and brush or watercolour pen

THERAPIST'S INSIGHT

Intentional breathing engages the parasympathetic nervous system, helping to reduce stress responses and calming the mind. Combining the breath with brush strokes helps to centre attention more closely on the breath, which is particularly helpful at regulating emotions and regaining focus for those with ADHD.

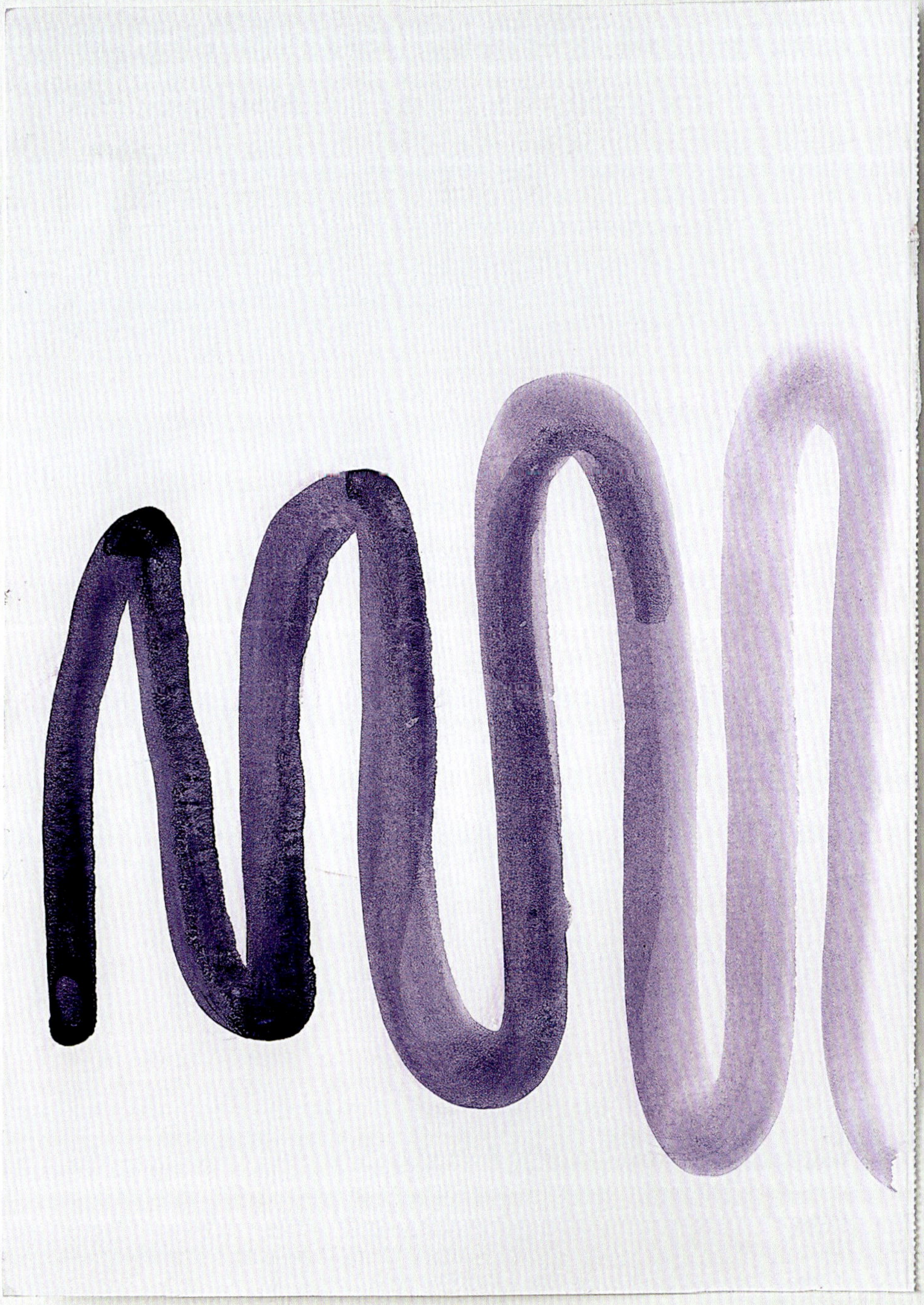

EXERCISE 3

Weighted colour wash

Large, sweeping movements encourage relaxation and emotional regulation. Colour washes mimic the comforting feeling of being wrapped or held, which can help ease anxiety and sensory overload.

INSTRUCTIONS

1. Use a clean, wet brush to lightly wet the whole page. Sweep the brush across the paper.
2. Choose a calming colour (for example: blue, lavender, sage).
3. Add paint to your brush and sweep the brush across the page in broad strokes.
4. Add additional calming colours in a second wash, if you like.
5. Pause and imagine the colour settling over you like a soft blanket.

WHAT YOU NEED

- ⇛ Watercolour paper
- ⇛ Large brush
- ⇛ Watercolours

THERAPIST'S INSIGHT

The movements in this exercise engage the body and senses, creating a somatic experience. This activates neural pathways, helping the brain form new connections and respond in different ways.

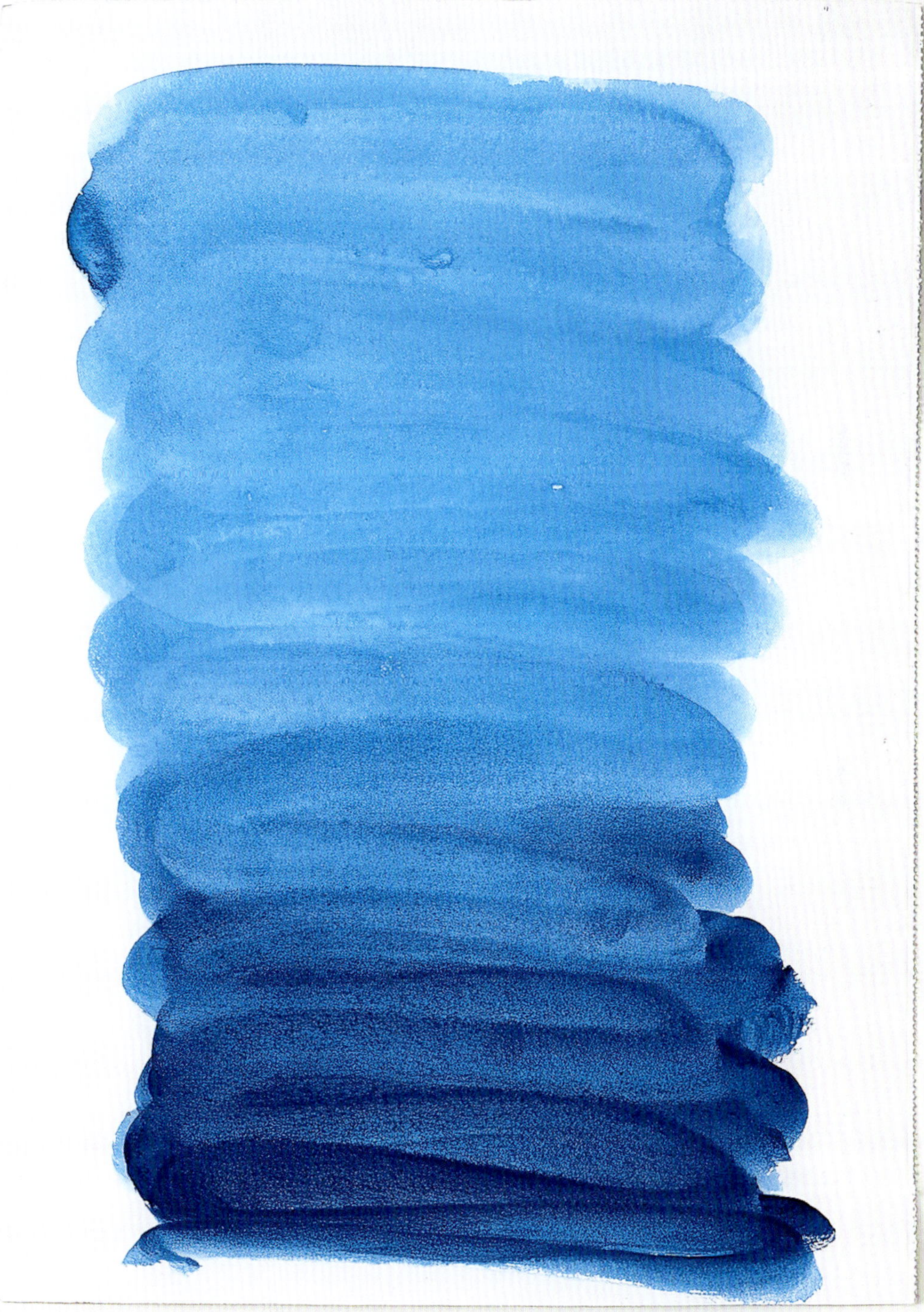

EXERCISE 4

Circles of safety

Repetition and round shapes naturally soothe the nervous system. The circle becomes a visual symbol of safety, containment and gentle expansion.

INSTRUCTIONS

1. Draw circles that overlap.
2. Move at a pace that feels calm, not rushed.
3. Stop when the page feels complete.
4. Colour the spaces created where the circles overlap. Use colours that make you feel calm.
5. If the outlines of the circles become unclear, feel free to retrace over them with a darker pen to make them more visible again.
6. Fill the shapes with simple, calming patterns using a fineliner pen, if you like.

WHAT YOU NEED

⇛ Paper

⇛ Pen, pencil or acrylic marker, in colours you like

⇛ Fineliner (optional)

THERAPIST'S INSIGHT

Research shows that doodling in or around a circle boosts blood flow to the brain's reward pathway, more than free drawing. When life feels chaotic, circles help contain the noise and calm your mind.

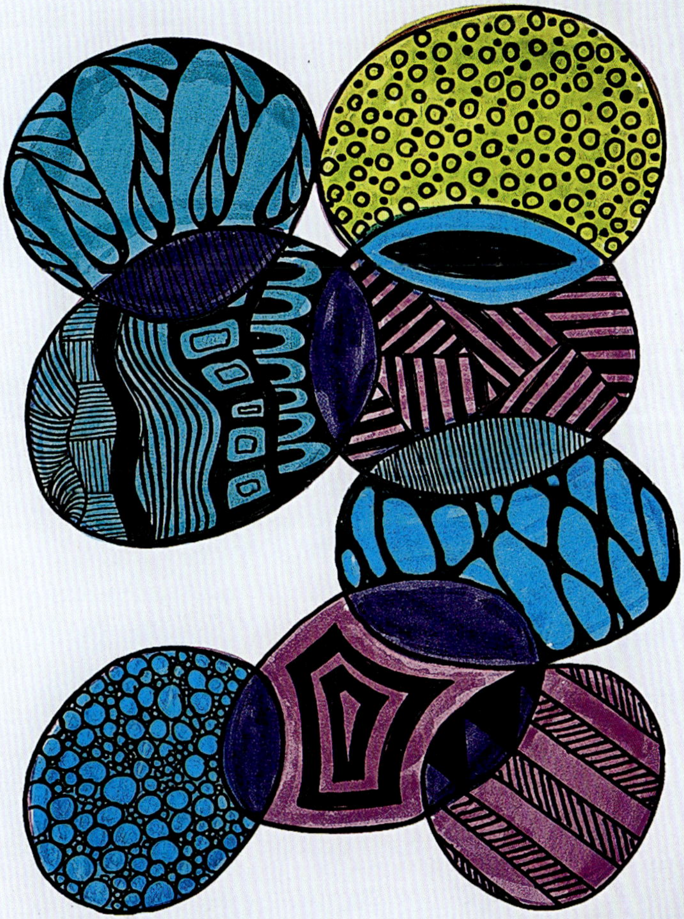

EXERCISE 5

Tracing hands

Tracing your hand reconnects you to your body and brings your attention to what you can feel. Decorating within the shape encourages a gentle, focused attention on the page.

INSTRUCTIONS

1. Place one hand on the paper.
2. Slowly trace around your fingers and palm with the pencil or pen.
3. Fill the inside of the hand with patterns, shapes or colours. For an added sensory experience you can glue scrap material inside the shape to make a collage.
4. Repeat with the other hand, if you like.
5. Enjoy the process.

WHAT YOU NEED

- → Paper
- → Pencil or pen
- → Glue and scrap material (optional)

THERAPIST'S INSIGHT

The feeling of the paper beneath your fingers and the marker brushing along your hand creates a sensory connection that helps you ground yourself. It is a gentle reminder that you are here in this moment, fully present.

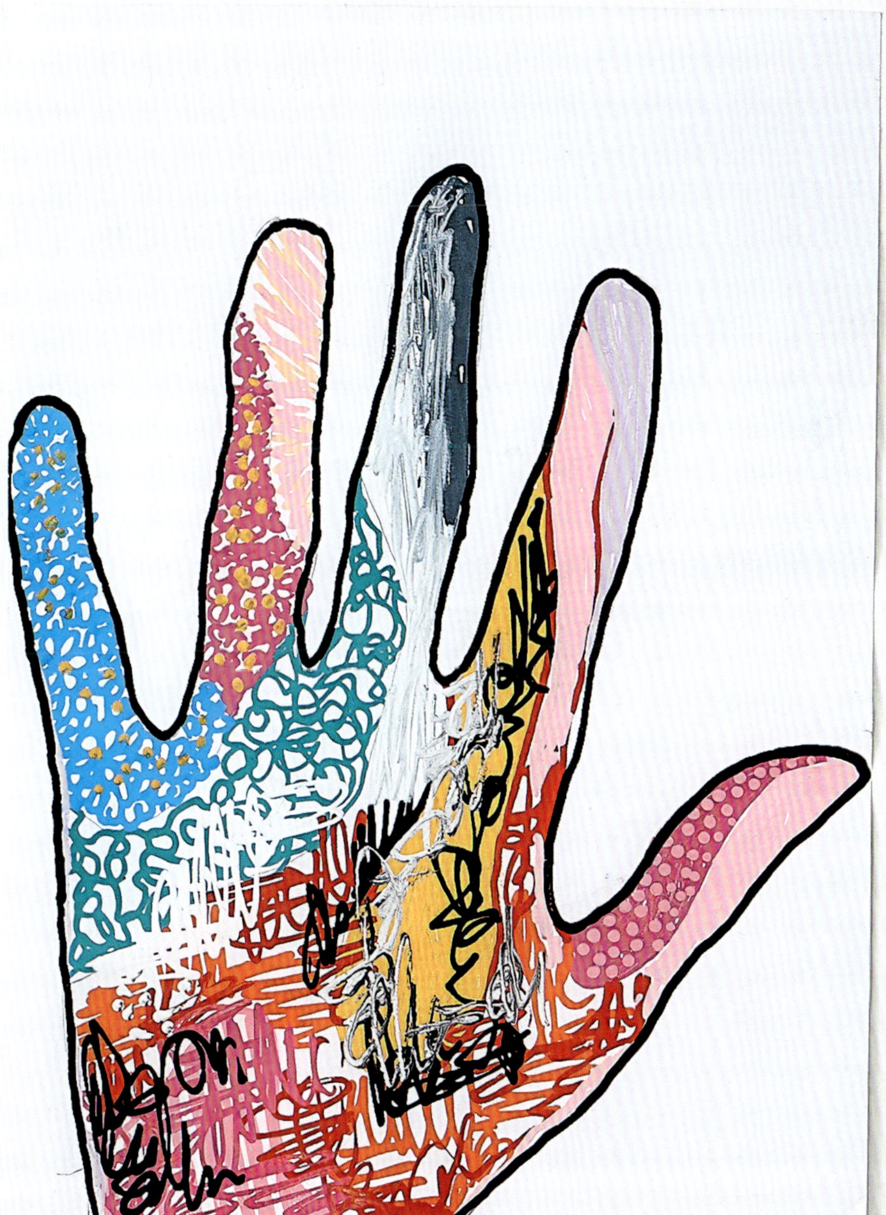

EXERCISE 6

Bilateral drawing

Bilateral drawing is a simple, non-verbal creative activity that many neurodivergent people find supportive. Using both hands at the same time in a left–right rhythm can help the body and brain settle. This kind of movement may support nervous-system regulation, help the two sides of the brain work together, and make it easier to focus or process feelings – without needing words.

You don't need to do this 'right'. Go at your own pace and notice what feels comfortable for you.

WHAT YOU NEED

- ⇛ Paper or card (A4 or larger is ideal)
- ⇛ Two pens/pencils/markers in different colours (ideally those that make the same kind of mark)

INSTRUCTIONS

1. Sit at a table with a piece of paper or card in front of you. Draw a centre line, or fold the paper or card in half to create one then open it out.
2. Hold a pen or pencil in each hand.

THERAPIST'S INSIGHT

Drawing with both hands works like a stim, helping you manage your sensory overload. Just as rocking or fidgeting can calm the nervous system, bilateral drawing gives structured sensory input that supports focus and reduces overwhelm.

3. Place both hands in the middle of the page.
   Then start drawing circles outwards:
   - The left hand draws a circle to the left.
   - The right hand draws a circle to the right.

   Don't worry if the circles are not perfect. It's about the movement, not the result.

4. Try to keep the circles moving together, slowly and smoothly. The symmetry can feel deeply satisfying for pattern-loving brains. Moving both hands together helps your body feel safe and settled, a bit like walking or rocking.

5. Breathe while you draw.

6. Reverse the direction of your hands, if you like.

7. You can do this exercise with music, or with your eyes closed if you want to explore the experience more fully.

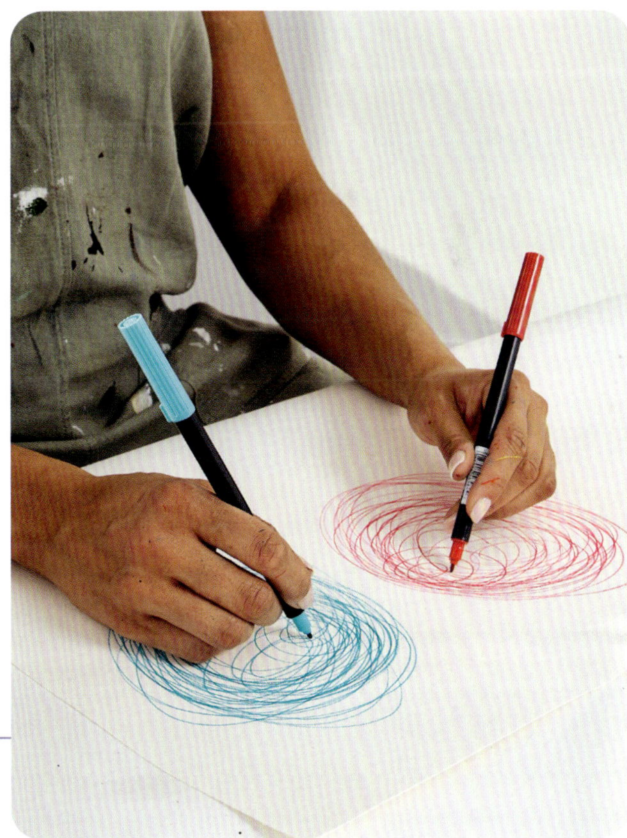

AFFIRMATION
Presence is enough.

EXERCISE 7

Colour breathing

Associating colour with breathing deepens awareness and calms your body. It turns breathing into something visual and rhythmic.

INSTRUCTIONS

1. Choose a colour that matches how you feel.
2. As your breathe in, draw a stroke or shape.
3. As you breathe out, repeat.
4. Continue until the page feels full, or your breath feels softer.
5. If you like, now fill the shapes with more patterns, lines or colours.

WHAT YOU NEED

⇛ Paper

⇛ Any colouring tool for drawing

THERAPIST'S INSIGHT

This exercise mirrors box breathing, where you breathe in for 4 seconds, hold your breath for 4 seconds, then breathe out for 4 seconds. Try combining the exercise with this breathing pattern to really maximize the calming benefits.

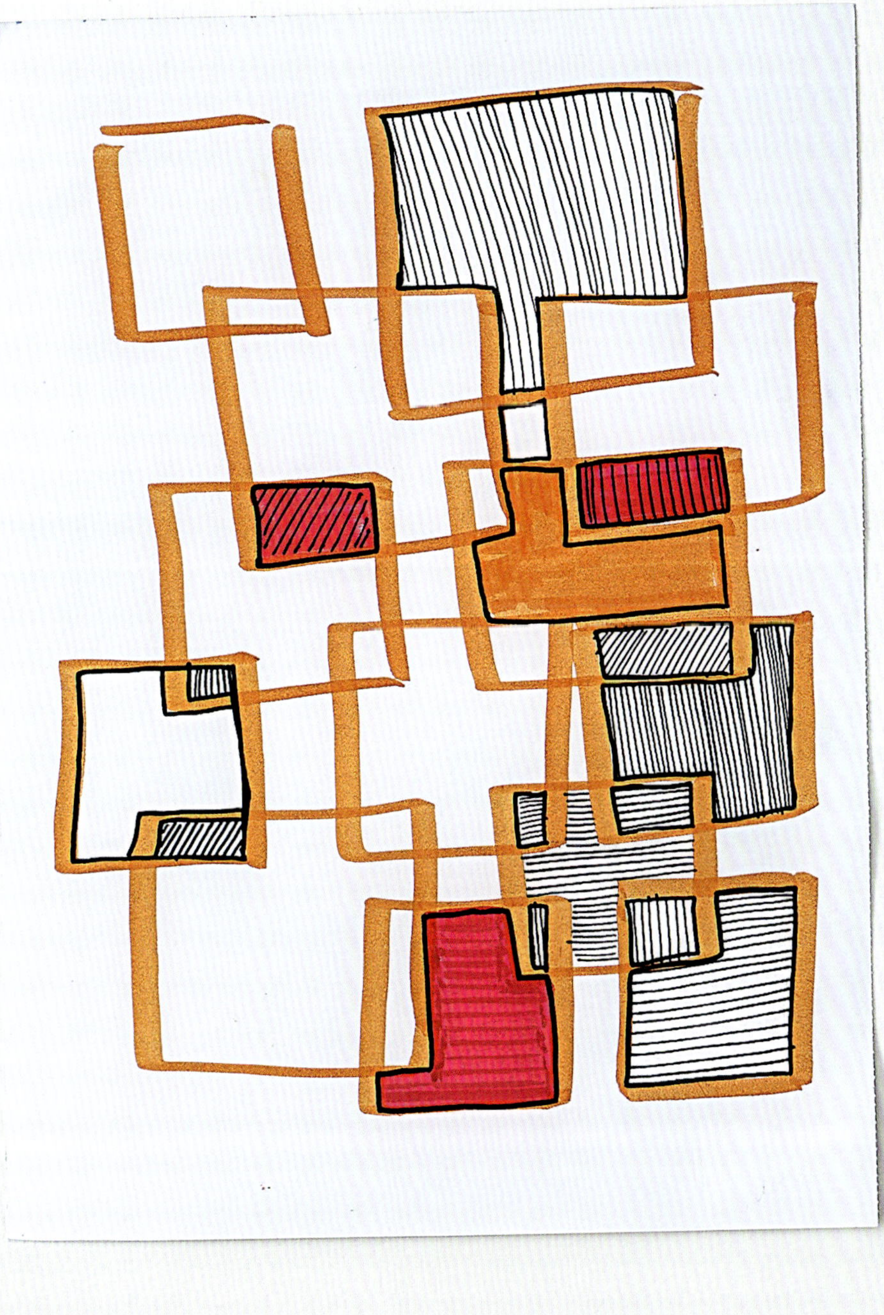

EXERCISE 8

Soothing symmetry

Making mirrored shapes can create a sense of balance and predictability. The fold-and-press method removes the pressure to be perfect and can help you feel more relaxed.

WHAT YOU NEED

⇒ Paper

⇒ Paint and brush or ink and dropper

INSTRUCTIONS

1. Fold the paper in half and unfold it.
2. Paint shapes, or use ink drops to create them, on one half of the paper only.
3. Fold the paper in half to transfer the shapes while the paint or ink is still wet.
4. Unfold the paper and observe the symmetry.
5. Add small details if it feels calming.

THERAPIST'S INSIGHT

Anxiety often comes from the fear of the unknown. Accepting the uncertainty in this exercise – not knowing how the paint will behave – mirrors our acceptance of future possibilities.

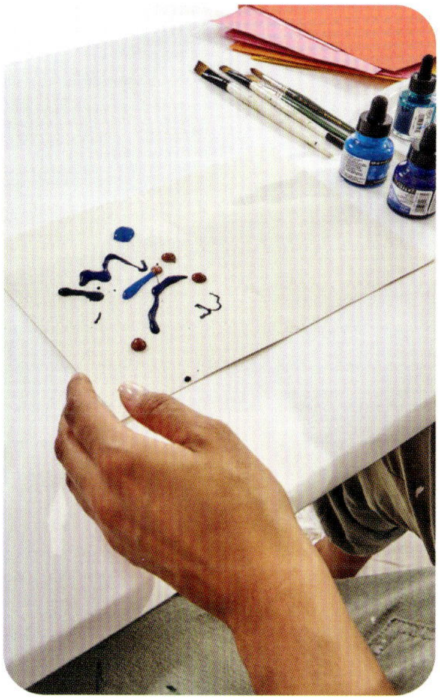

Step 2

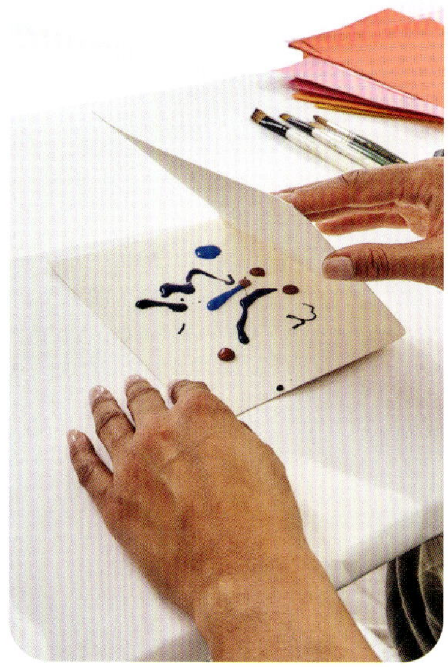

Step 3

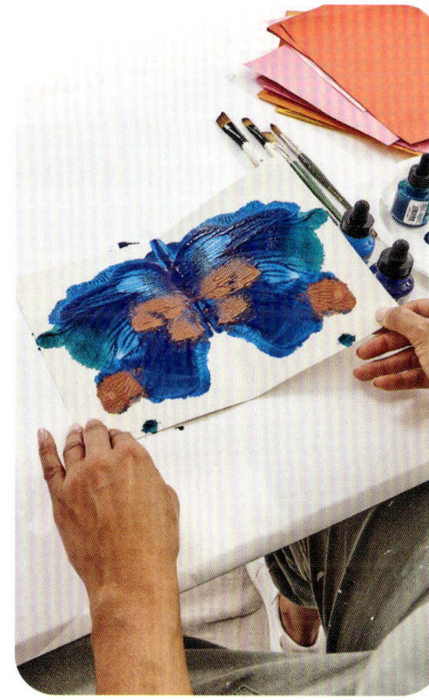

Step 4

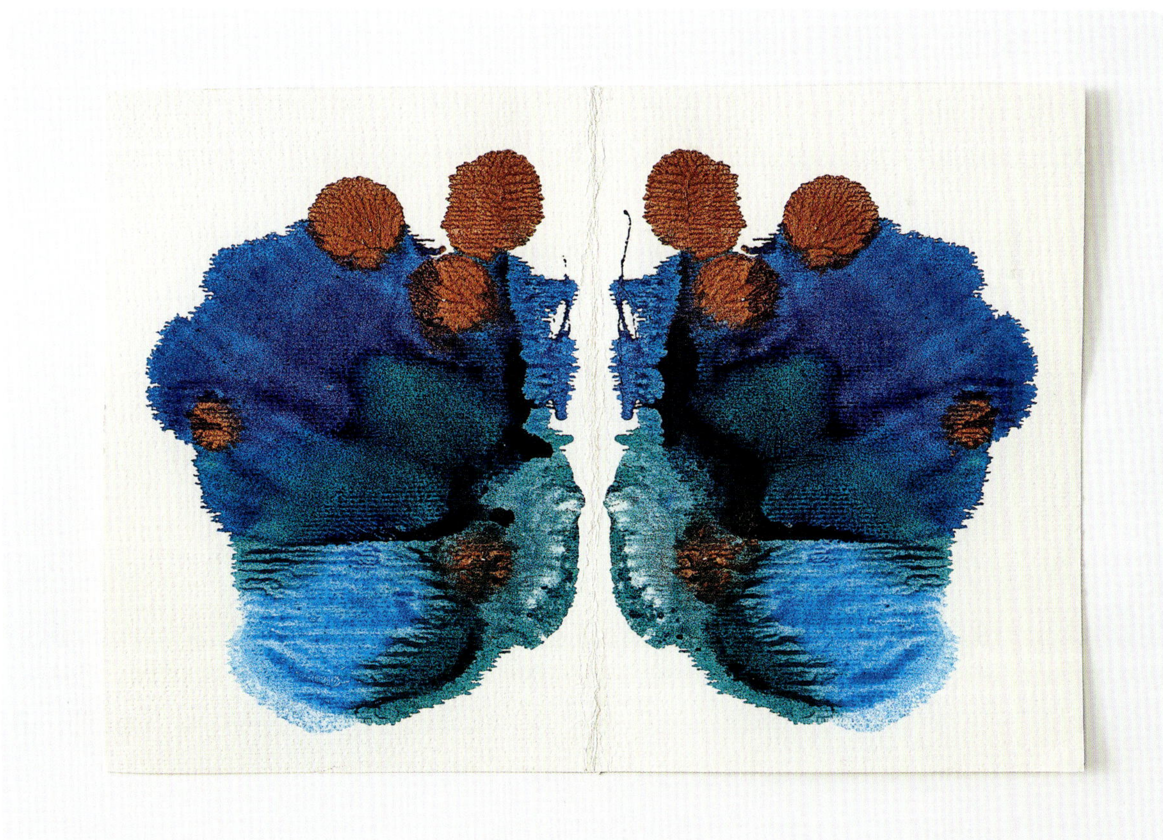

EXERCISE 9

Scribble release

Fast scribbling can release stored tension. Moving more slowly afterwards supports self-regulation and emotional grounding.

INSTRUCTIONS

1. Set a timer for 1 minute.
2. Scribble quickly and freely on your paper.
3. When the timer stops, pause.
4. Look for the shapes or softer forms in the scribble.
5. Gently refine or decorate these shapes. Fill in the spaces created during the scribbling with colour or patterns.

WHAT YOU NEED

- Paper
- Pen, pencil or crayon
- Timer

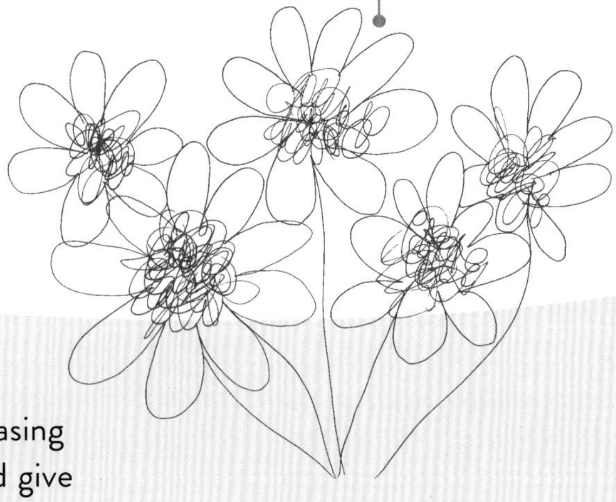

Alternative drawing

THERAPIST'S INSIGHT

Our bodies store stress, and if this isn't released, it can create physical and mental tension. By releasing this tension, you reduce your stress hormones and give yourself more resilience to cope with future stresses.

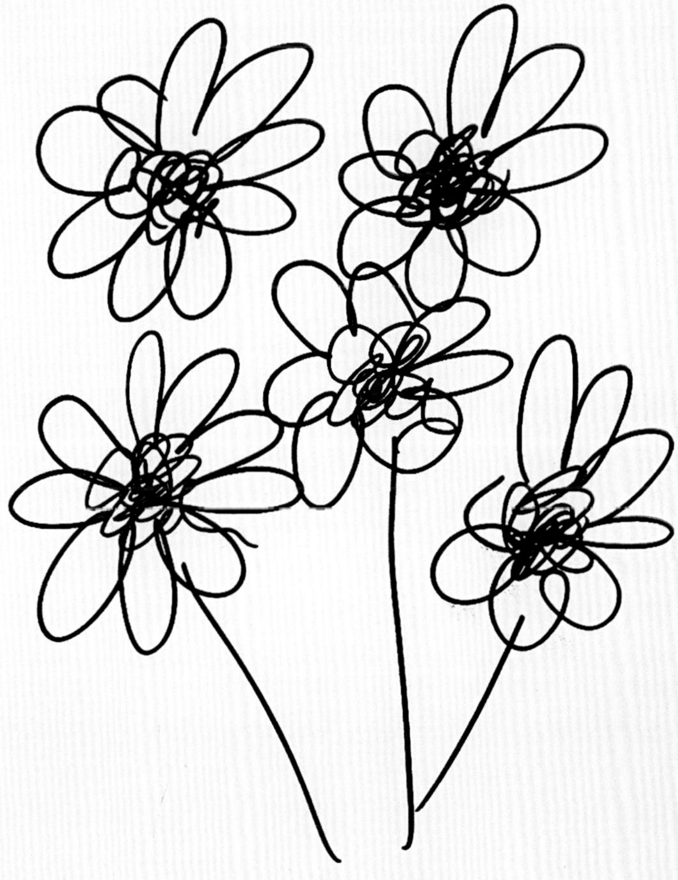

EXERCISE 10

Paint with texture

Notice how the raised surfaces and textures in this exercise feel, and how the light affects them. This calming sensory experience connects you to the present moment.

INSTRUCTIONS

1. Mix acrylic paint with your choice of these everyday materials:
   - ⇛ Salt (for a grainy effect)
   - ⇛ Sand (for organic grit)
   - ⇛ Flour or baking soda (for a softer texture)
   - ⇛ Tissue paper (for irregular bumps).
2. Apply the paint to the board or card using a brush, palette knife, sponge or your fingers.
3. Once dry, lightly brush paint in the same or a different colour across the surface. The raised areas will pick up the colour of the paint.

WHAT YOU NEED

- ⇛ Canvas board or card
- ⇛ Acrylic paint and brush
- ⇛ An everyday material of your choice to create texture
- ⇛ Palette knife (optional)
- ⇛ Sponge (optional)

THERAPIST'S INSIGHT

Touching different textures grounds your body and senses, helping the brain feel reward and relief. As feelings of overwhelm decrease, the prefrontal cortex works more effectively, helping you to organize your thoughts more easily.

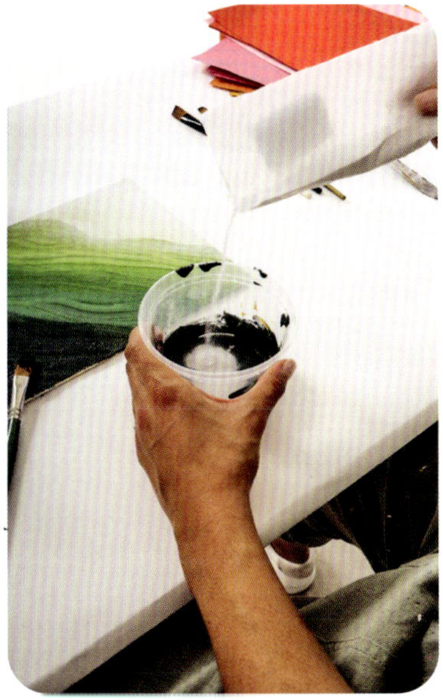

Step 1

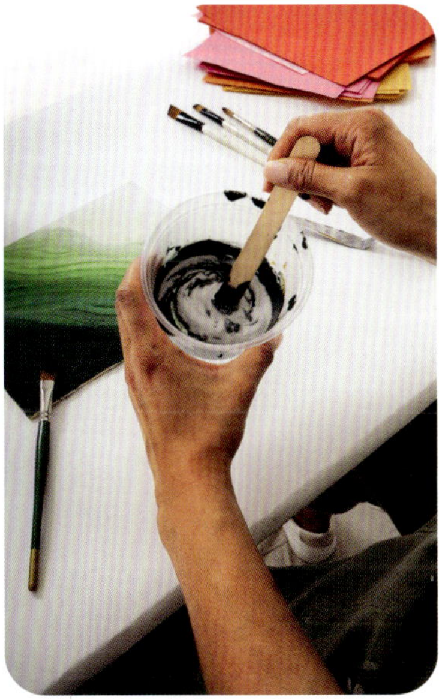

Step 2

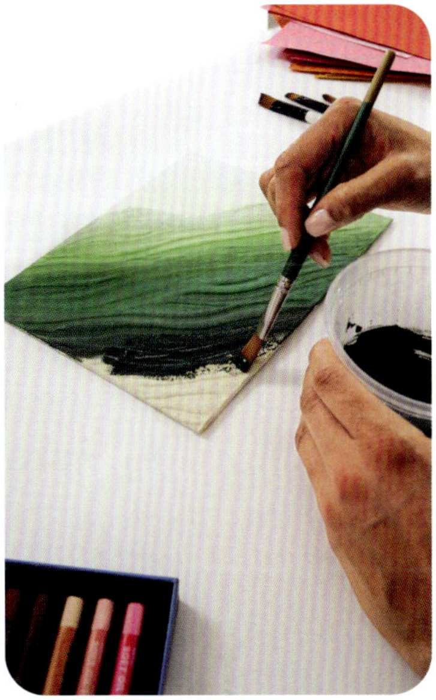

Step 3

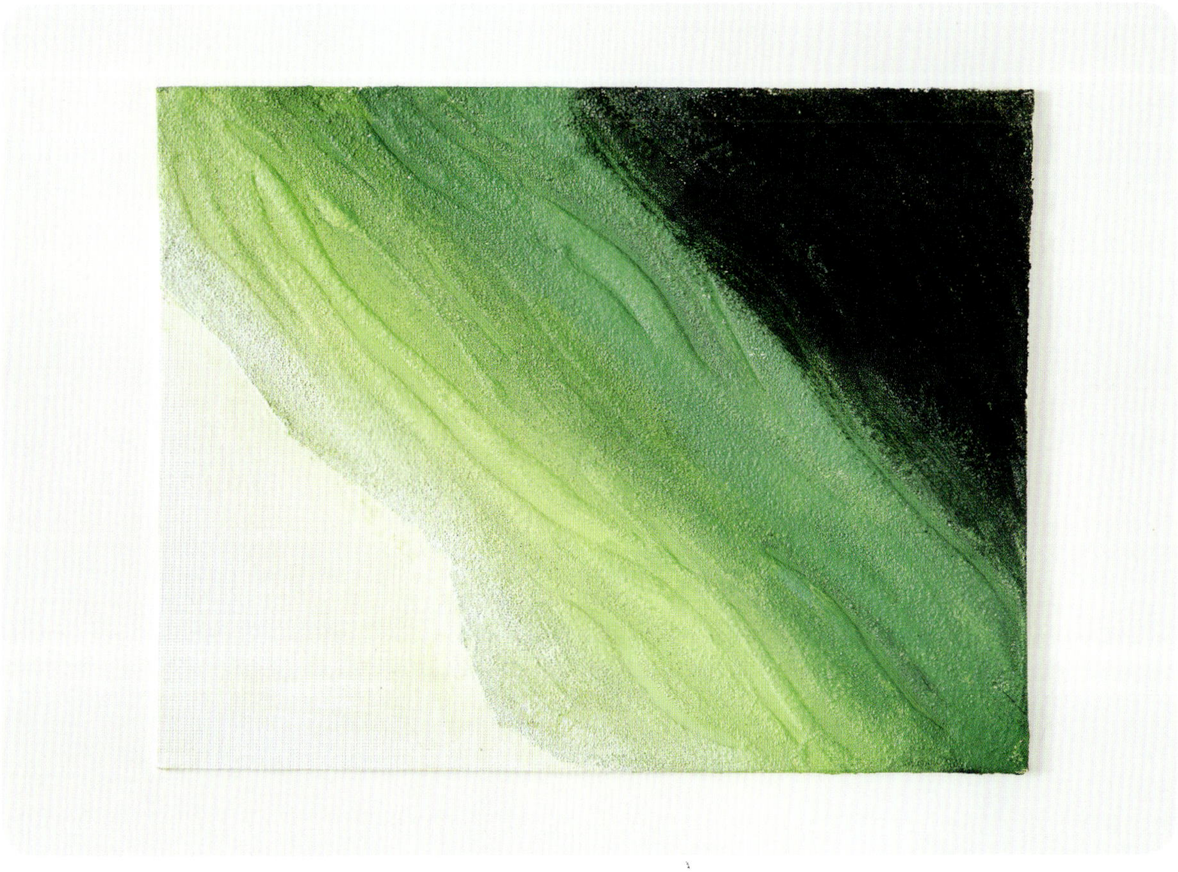

CHAPTER 2

RELEASING ANXIETY

Introduction

Anxiety often shows up in the body before we can put it into words. It can feel like tight muscles, restlessness, looping thoughts or a constant sense of being 'on alert'. For neurodivergent minds, especially, anxiety can build quietly over time. It is often linked to sensory overload, masking, uncertainty, or living in a world that asks a lot.

This chapter offers creative practices that are designed to help release some of that held tension in a gentle, non-confrontational way. The exercises focus on movement, repetition and containment. They give the nervous system somewhere safe to direct its energy, allowing anxiety to soften through doing rather than thinking.

There is no requirement to name your anxiety or understand where it comes from. You do not need to explain it, justify it or fix it.

As you move through this chapter, pay attention to small shifts. A deeper breath. A slower pace. A sense of relief or release, even if it's brief. These moments matter.

This chapter is not about eliminating anxiety altogether.

It simply shows you how creativity can provide a steady, compassionate outlet when your mind feels full.

THERAPIST'S NOTE

Releasing anxiety can be difficult because holding anxious feelings can feel like a form of protection. For some anxiety is always present, while for others it creeps in when you least expect it.

These exercises help you release anxiety and become more aware of yourself in the moment. They work by creating a sense of safety within the nervous system, which helps lower the stress response. When the parasympathetic nervous system – our 'rest and digest' state – is activated, the brain senses safety. Staying in this state allows the body's energy to settle, easing the need to stay on high alert.

EXERCISE 11

Storm to stillness

Anxiety can create an internal 'storm' – your thoughts feel fast and tangled and your body feels tense. This exercise teaches your body how to shift from chaos to calm.

INSTRUCTIONS

1. Start by drawing quick, chaotic scribbles or overlapping lines in pen or pencil. Do not control them – let the movement express any tension.
2. Fill the shapes created by the overlapping lines with more scribbles to release extra tension then pause. Take one slow breath.
3. Choose a soft-coloured marker or paint, and draw or paint around each scribble with smooth, calming strokes.
4. Retrace your original lines with a calming colour. Continue until the page feels calmer.

WHAT YOU NEED

⇛ Paper

⇛ Pen or pencil

⇛ Coloured markers or paint and brush

⇛ Coloured pencils

AFFIRMATION

The storm does not stay for ever.

THERAPIST'S INSIGHT

Using free, energetic marks at the start of this exercise helps to neutralize and clear any troubling feelings. This allows your mind and body to return to a state of calm and rest.

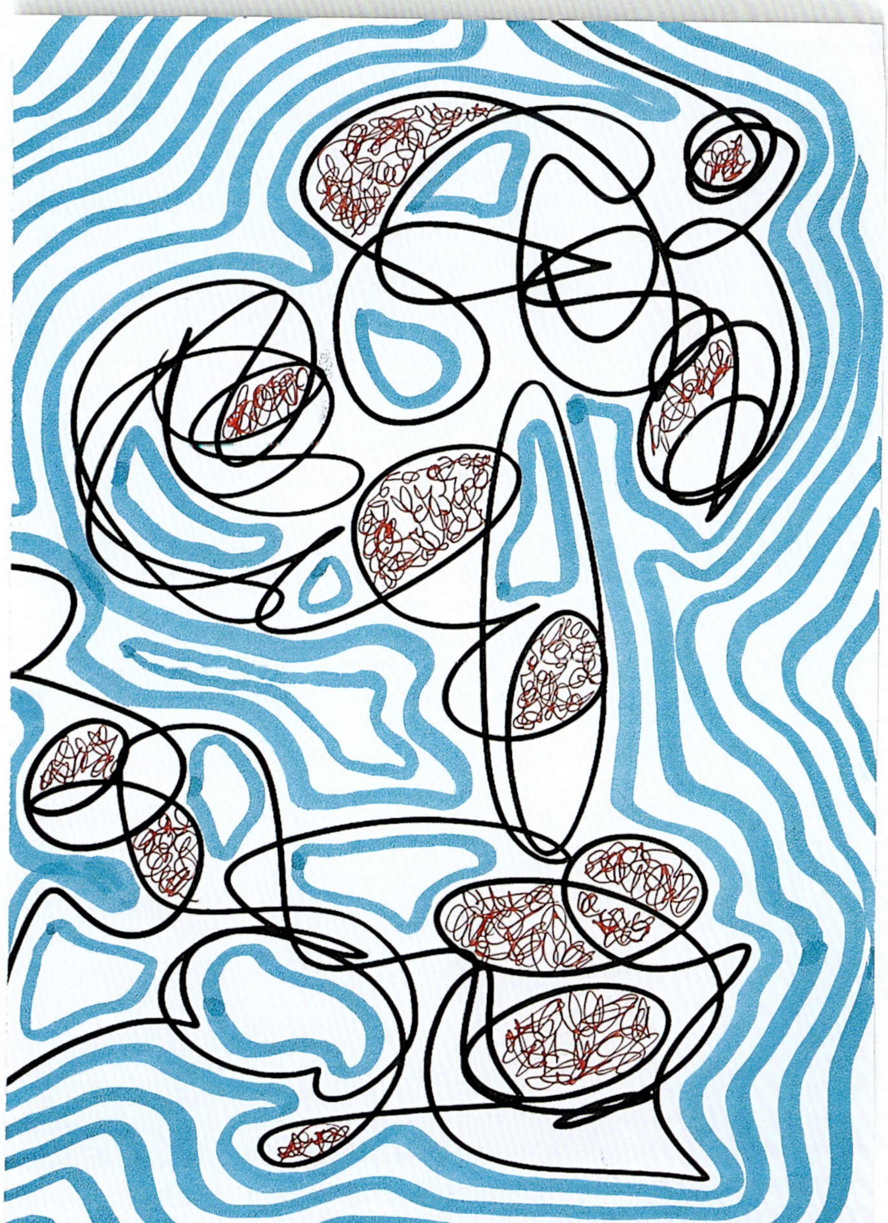

EXERCISE 12

Anxiety box

Containing worry visually in a box helps the mind feel safer. If you transform the outside of the box into something calming, the experience of anxiety can be rewired – feelings of overwhelm can be held and managed.

INSTRUCTIONS

1. Draw a box in the centre of the page.
2. Fill the inside with messy lines, words or marks representing anxious thoughts.
3. Close the box by drawing a firm border around it.
4. Decorate the outside of the box with soft, soothing colours or patterns.
5. Spend time with the outer calming patterns, rather than with what is on the inside.

WHAT YOU NEED

⇛ Paper

⇛ Pen or markers

THERAPIST'S INSIGHT

Placing our anxieties in a contained space helps us separate anxious thoughts from our sense of self. In this way you can view them as something outside of you, making them feel more manageable and less consuming.

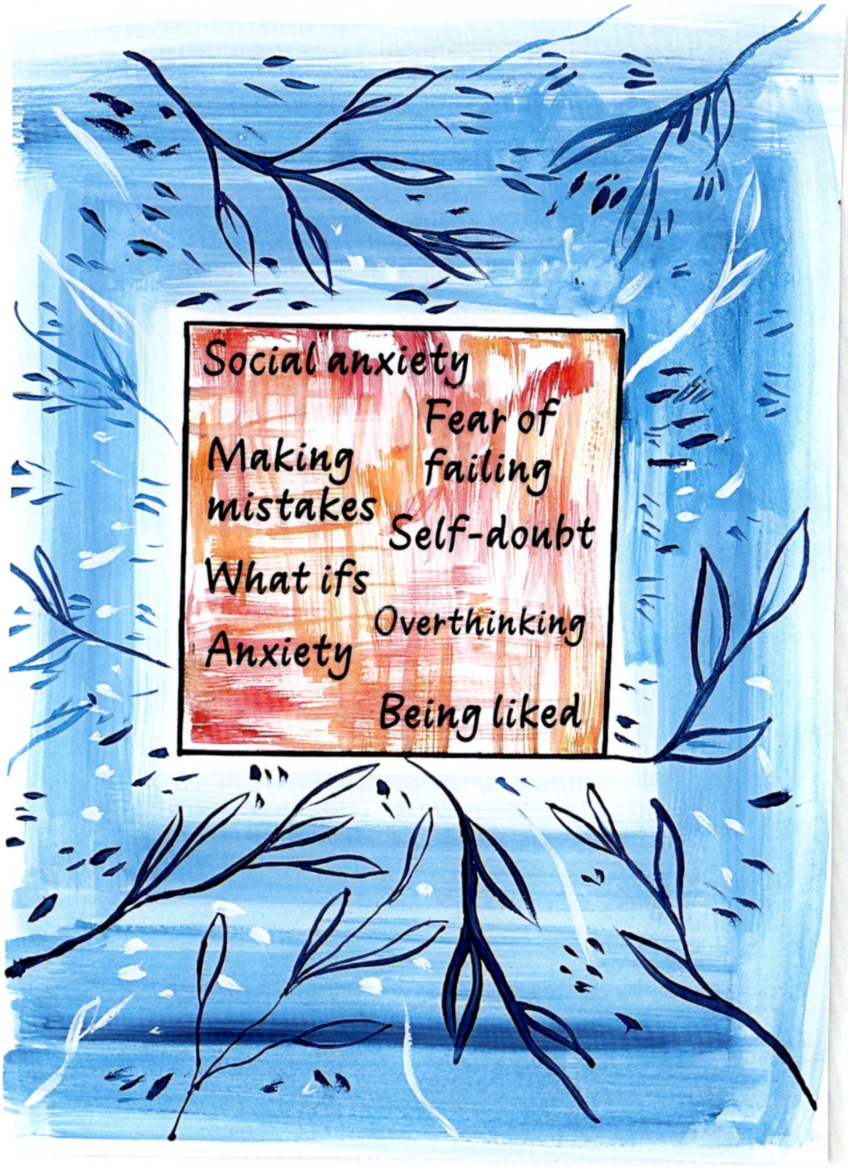
Social anxiety
Fear of failing
Making mistakes
Self-doubt
What ifs
Overthinking
Anxiety
Being liked

EXERCISE 13

Tear & transform

Tearing paper can help release stored frustration or panic. Reassembling the pieces can feel empowering, showing that what feels broken can be shaped into something meaningful.

INSTRUCTIONS

1. Take a piece of scrap paper and tear it into pieces. Use any sort of scrap paper you like, such as paper for recycling, cereal boxes or sweet wrappers.
2. Let the tearing be messy and instinctive.
3. Arrange the torn pieces on a new sheet of paper in any way that feels interesting.
4. Glue or tape the pieces down.
5. Add colour or line details in pen or pencil, if you like.

WHAT YOU NEED

⇛ Paper

⇛ Scrap paper

⇛ Glue or tape

⇛ Pens or pencils (optional)

THERAPIST'S INSIGHT

This exercise teaches us how to transform something negative into something beautiful. By building cognitive flexibility, we learn to reframe difficult thoughts or experiences into perspectives that feel more balanced and neutral.

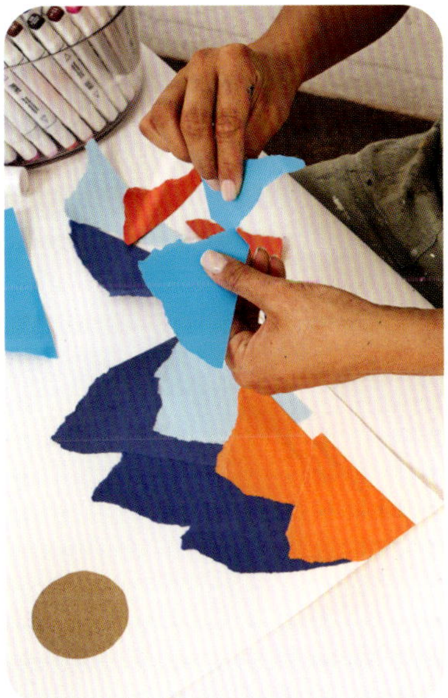

Step 2

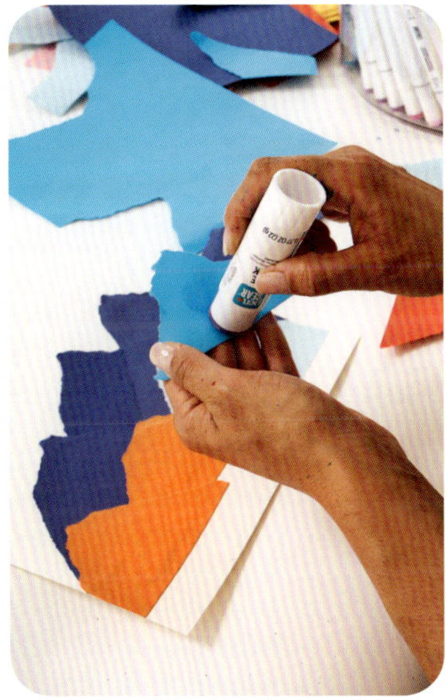

Step 3

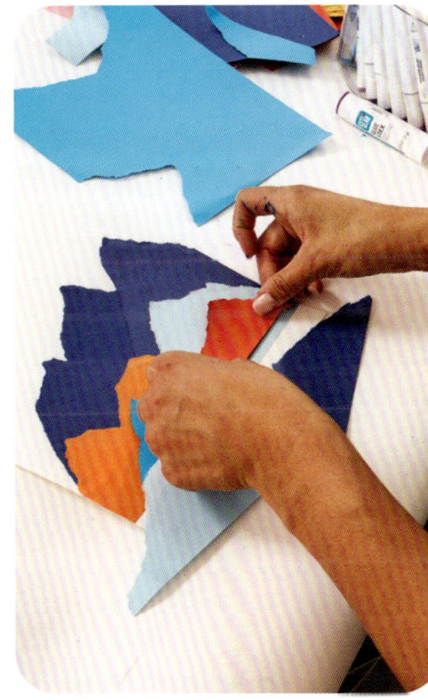

Step 4

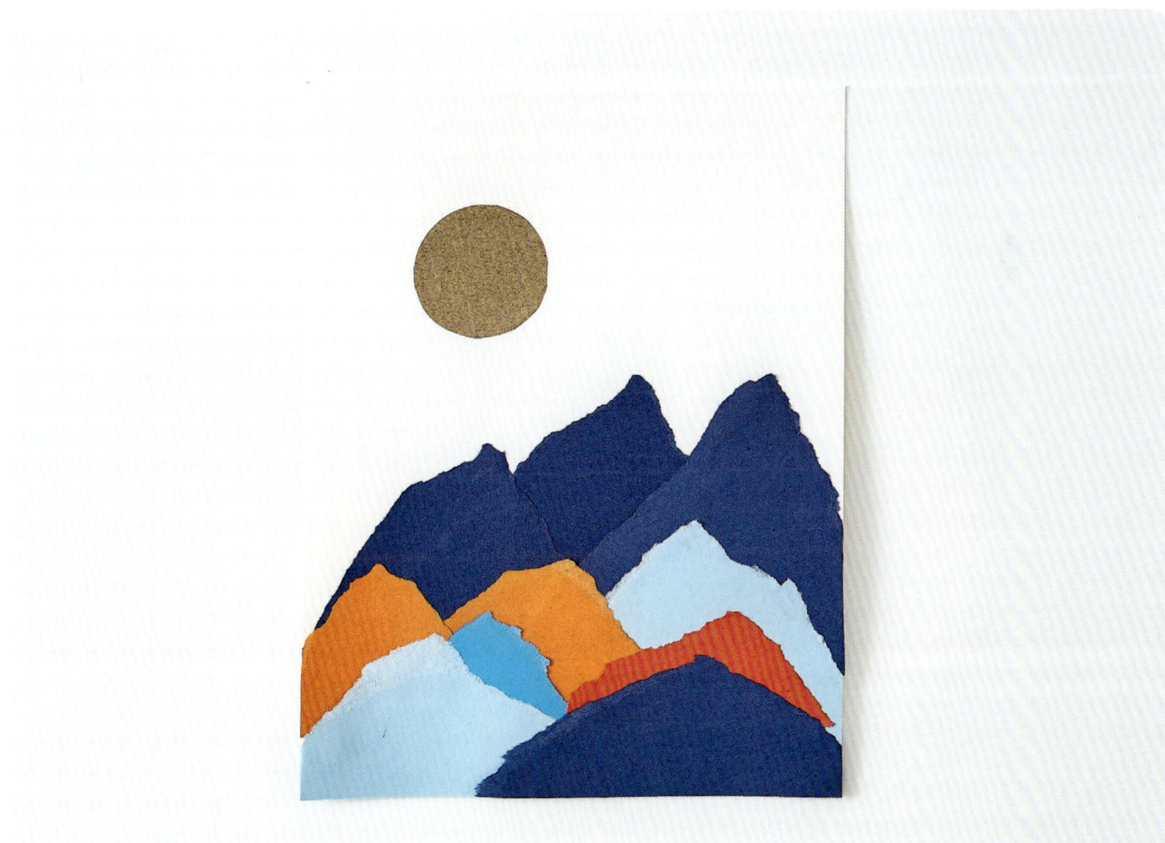

EXERCISE 14

Knot & untangle

Drawing knots represents how anxiety tangles your thoughts. Slowly softening and opening the lines mirrors the feeling of loosening internal tension.

INSTRUCTIONS

1. Draw looping, tangled knot shapes.
2. Let them overlap and twist – there is no need to plan.
3. Then choose one area and begin softening the lines into smooth curves.
4. In this way gradually 'untangle' the drawing section by section.
5. Continue until some areas feel open and spacious.

WHAT YOU NEED

⇒ Paper

⇒ Pens or pencils

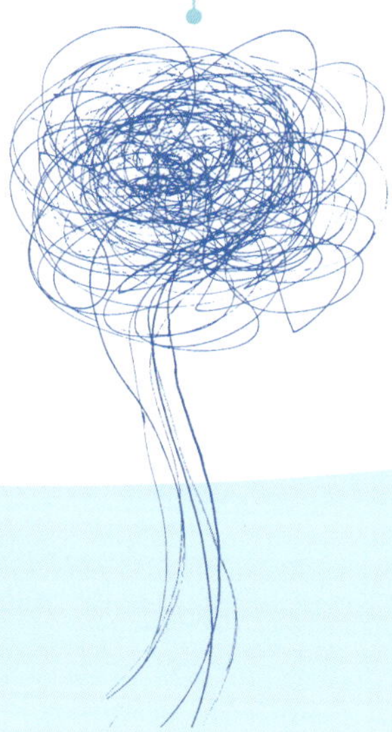

Alternative drawing

THERAPIST'S INSIGHT

When problems feel overwhelming and confusing, our emotions can feel tangled and knotted. Drawing knots helps release stored stress while giving us a sense of control as we untangle these emotions on the page.

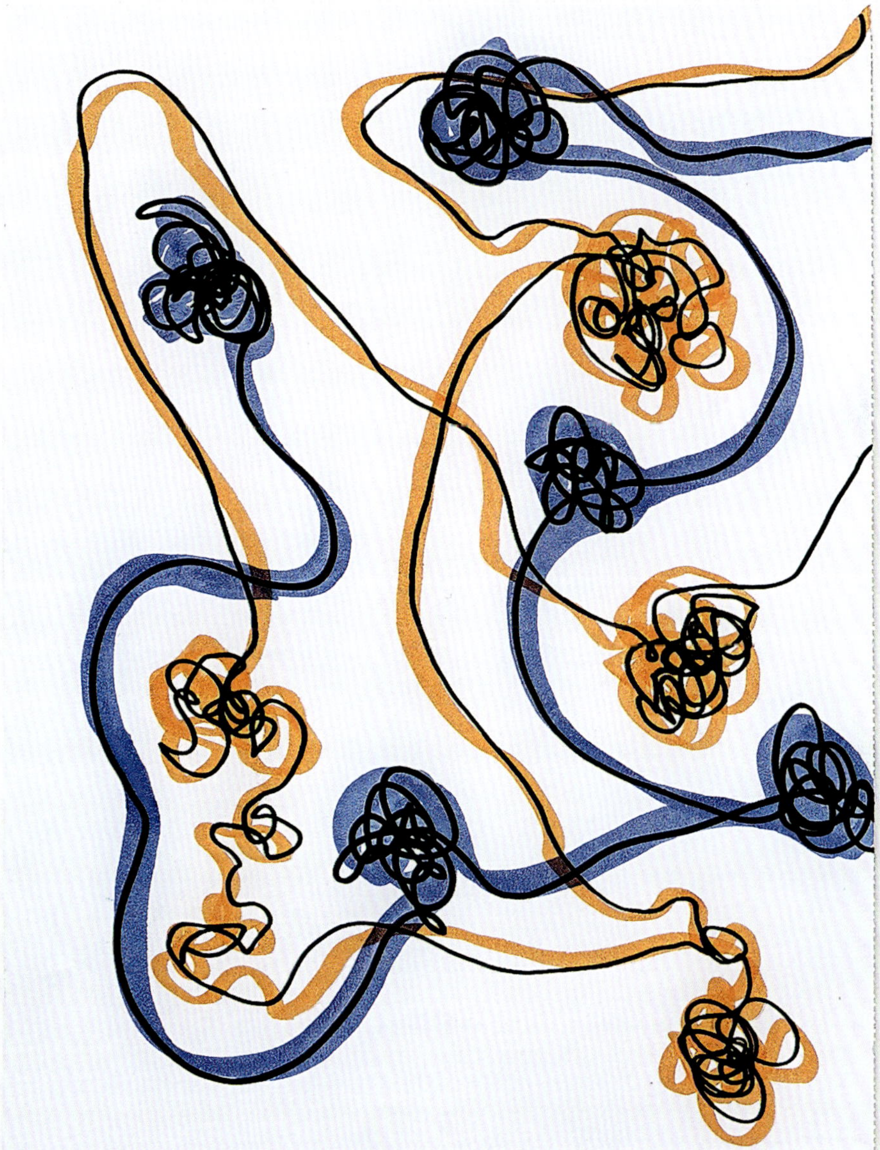

EXERCISE 15

Colour-mapping feelings

Externalizing feelings through colour reduces emotional overload. Putting feelings onto the page gives form to what seems invisible and overwhelming, and helps make them easier to see, understand and soothe.

INSTRUCTIONS

1. Choose colours that match the feelings you are experiencing right now.
2. Without planning, make marks, shapes or areas of colour on the page.
3. Let the colours overlap, mix or stand alone.
4. There is no right or wrong – this is expression, not art.
5. Stop when the feelings feel seen.

WHAT YOU NEED

⇛ Paper

⇛ Paints and brushes, markers and pencils in any colours

THERAPIST'S INSIGHT

Somatic body mapping is a therapeutic approach where a person draws their body and uses colour to show their emotions in different areas, helping make feelings visual. This exercise offers a similar experience, supporting you to identify and understand how you feel.

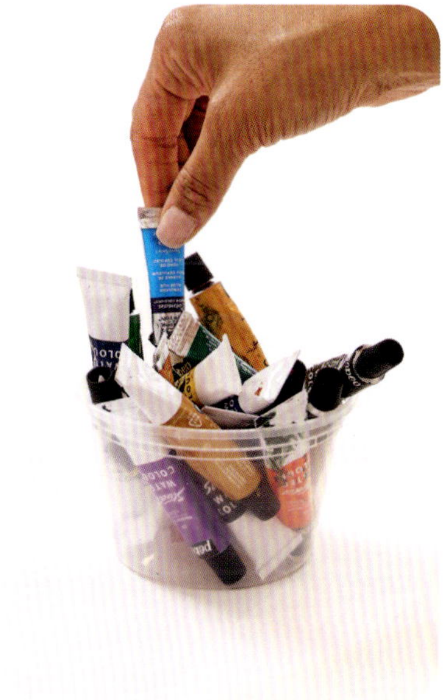

Step 2

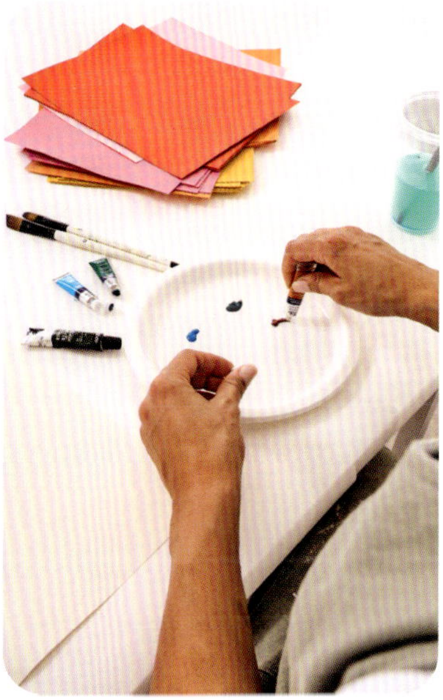

Step 3

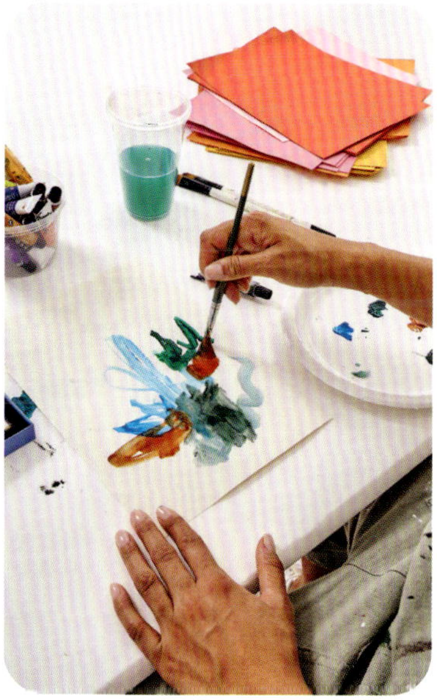

Step 4

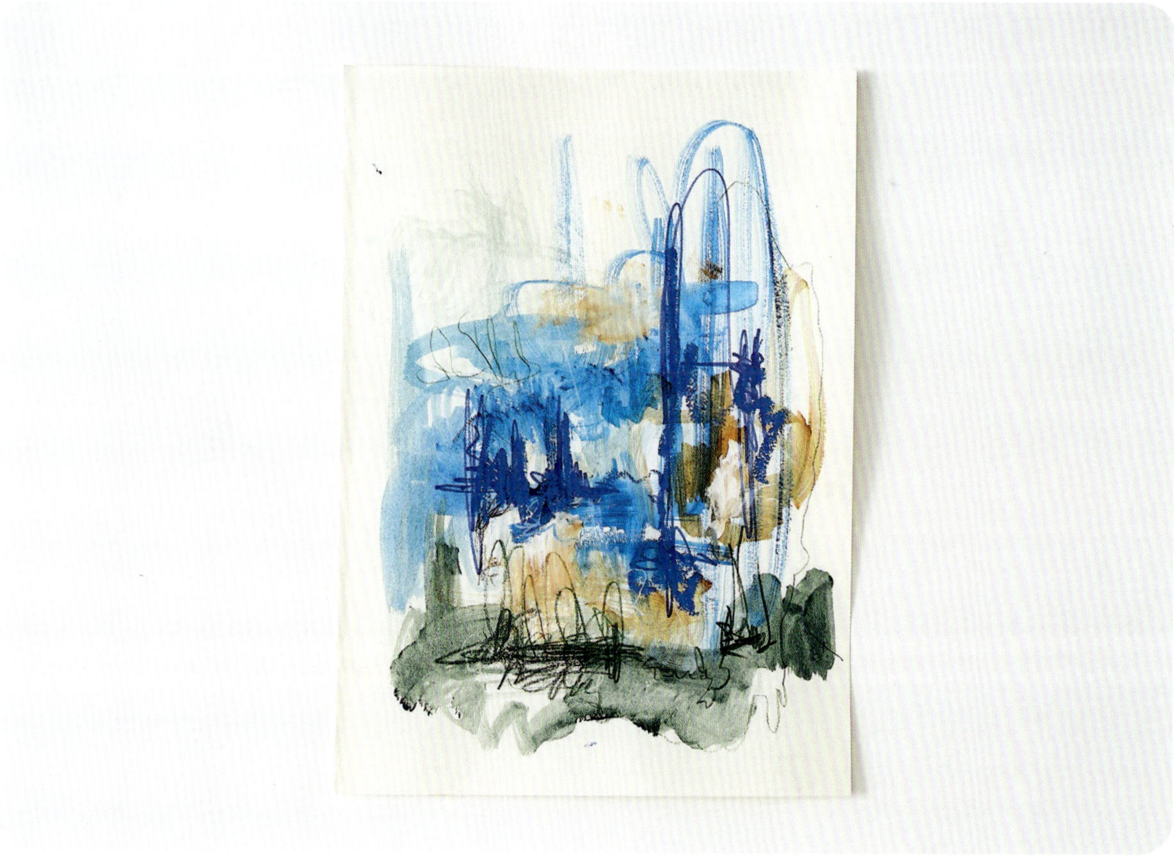

EXERCISE 16

Wave motion drawing

Drawing wave-like lines can mirror the natural rise and fall of anxious feelings. This can teach your nervous system that emotions come and go, rather than staying stuck.

INSTRUCTIONS

1. Begin drawing or painting wave shapes – rising, cresting and falling.
2. Let your hand move in long, continuous motions.
3. Vary the height and speed as feels most natural.
4. Continue until the movement feels smoother and quieter.
5. Notice the rhythmic flow that emerges.

WHAT YOU NEED

⇛ Paper

⇛ Pen, pencil or paint and brush

THERAPIST'S INSIGHT

Acceptance and Commitment Therapy (ACT) teaches us that emotions are transient. The wave drawing reflects this natural flow, reminding us that even difficult emotions rise, pass and move on.

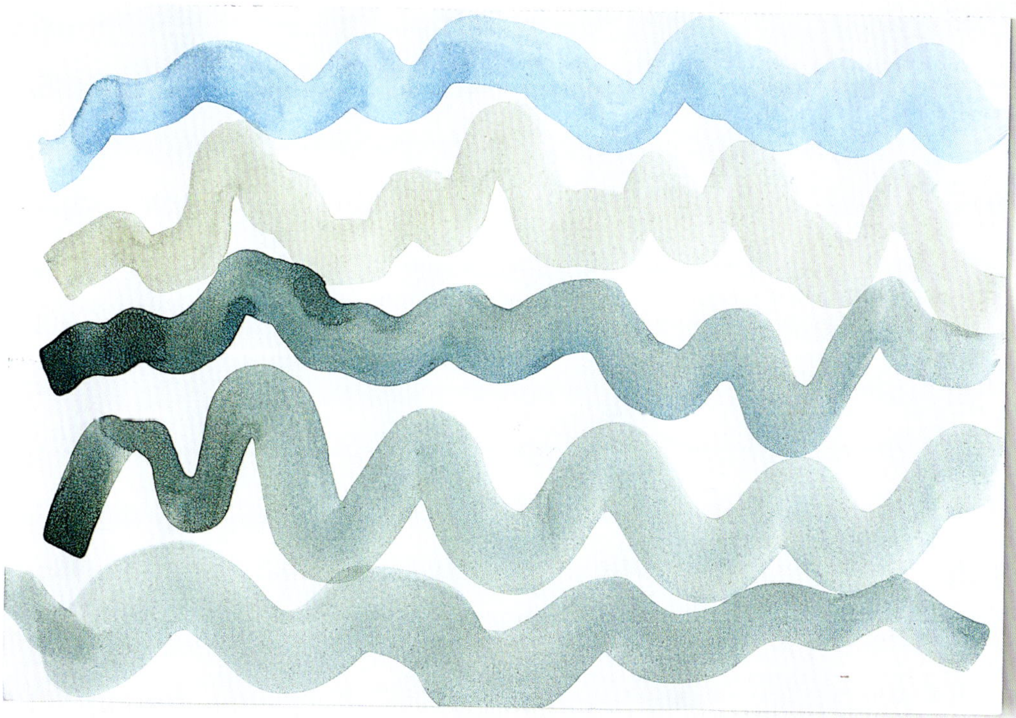

EXERCISE 17

Mindful mandalas

Repeatedly making the same patterns provides structure and safety. Mandalas naturally create a calming focus and help reduce mental spinning.

INSTRUCTIONS

1. Draw or trace a circle, using a compass if you wish.
2. Divide the circle into segments or simply begin adding patterns from the centre outwards.
3. Use repeated lines, shapes or dots.
4. Let your hand move slowly and rhythmically.
5. Continue until the pattern feels complete.

WHAT YOU NEED

⇛ Paper

⇛ Pen or coloured pens

⇛ Circular object to trace, or a compass (optional)

THERAPIST'S INSIGHT

Colouring in mandala shapes can activate both parts of the brain: the right hemisphere for colour selection and the left hemisphere for geometric patterns. Doing this can strengthen connections in the brain and reduce activity in the amygdala (see page 9), easing stress and anxiety.

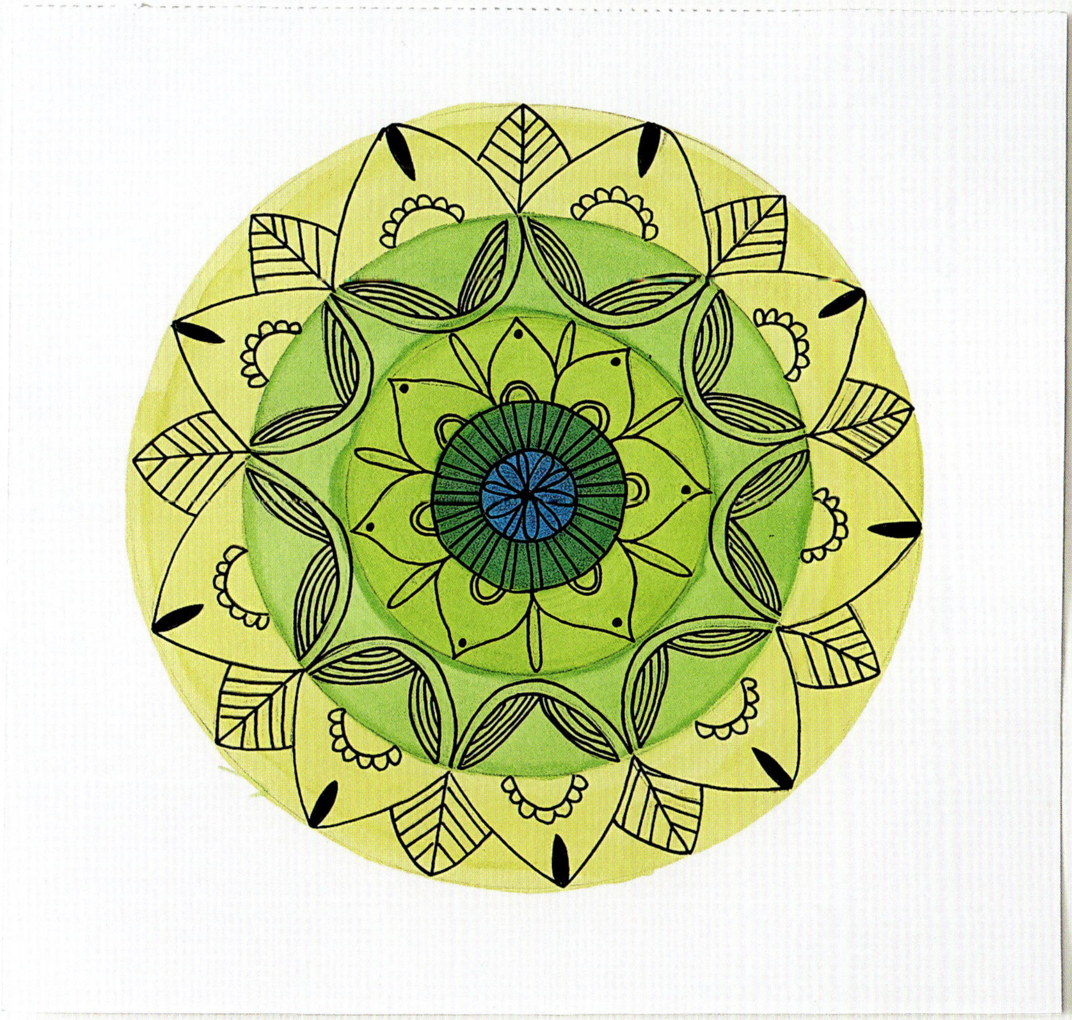

EXERCISE 18

Shatter & repair

This *kintsugi*-inspired exercise reminds us that being broken is not an ending. Repairing the piece helps you practise self-compassion and resilience.

INSTRUCTIONS

1. Draw a simple shape (a heart, bowl or circle).
2. Draw 'cracks' through the shape, to look like broken pottery.
3. Now trace over the cracks with gold or a bright, warm colour.
4. Add decorative marks, if you like.
5. Let it become something beautiful.

WHAT YOU NEED

⇛ Paper

⇛ Pencil or marker

⇛ Gold/bright pen or paint and brush

Kintsugi is the traditional Japanese art of mending broken pottery using a mixture of lacquer and a precious metal.

THERAPIST'S INSIGHT

Cognitive restructuring helps us reframe experiences and emotions, building resilience. This exercise reflects that process by transforming something broken into something new, reminding us that we continue to grow, evolve and learn.

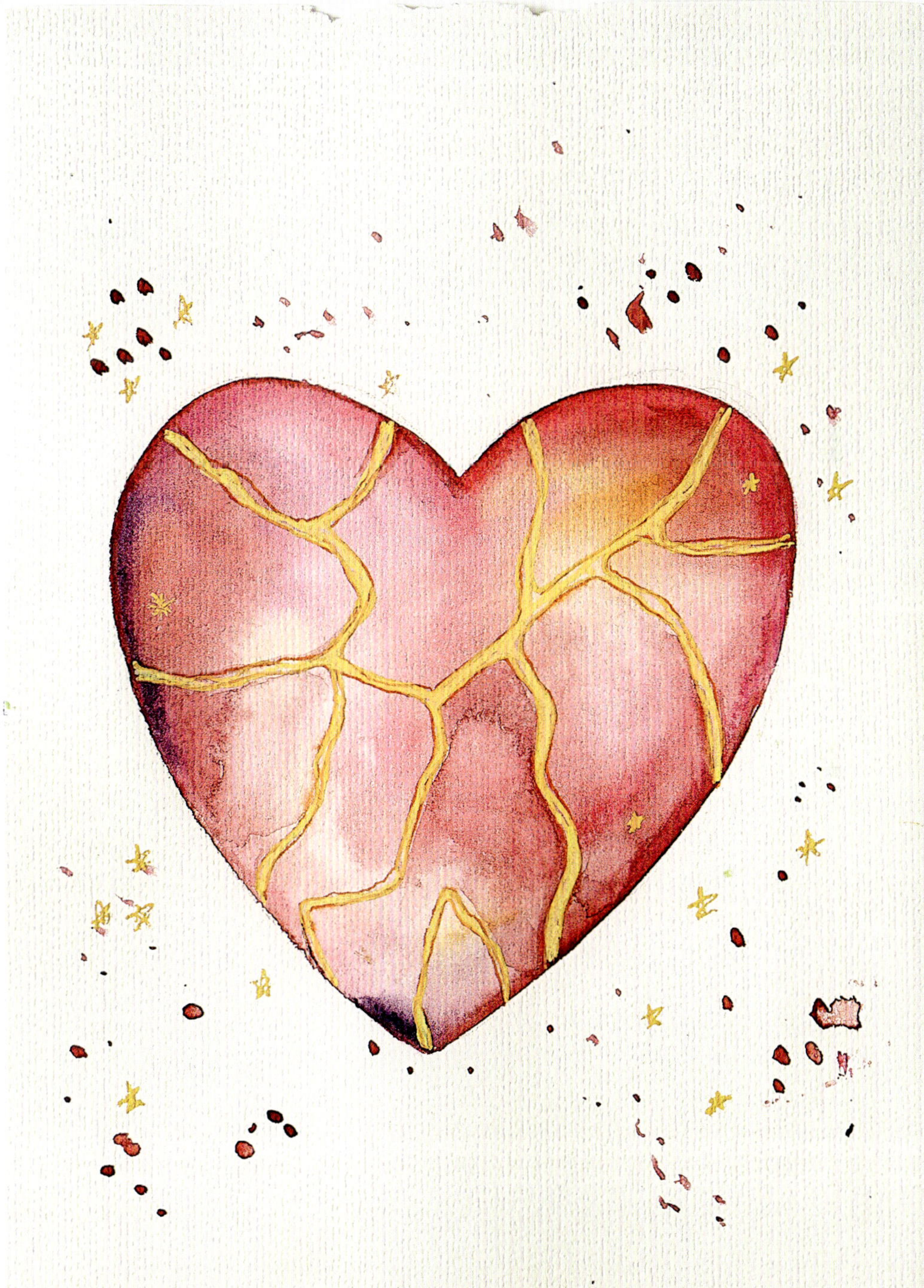

EXERCISE 19

Mindful dots

Making one dot for each breath is a simple grounding technique. It can help the nervous system slow down and interrupts anxious spirals.

INSTRUCTIONS

1. Take a slow breath in.
2. Place one dot on the paper as you breathe out.
3. Repeat at a gentle, unhurried pace.
4. Let the page fill slowly – there is no finish line.
5. Stop whenever your breath feels softer.

WHAT YOU NEED

⇛ Paper

⇛ Pen or marker

Another option is to use liquid paint in a bottle to create a textured dot effect. Carefully squeeze the bottle to release a dot onto the paper – this needs more hand–eye coordination and control.

THERAPIST'S INSIGHT

Breathing is one of the most effective ways to reduce anxiety. Slow, conscious breathing encourages a meditative state and supports the release of gamma-aminobutyric acid (GABA), a calming brain messenger that slows the nervous system, easing stress and supporting better sleep.

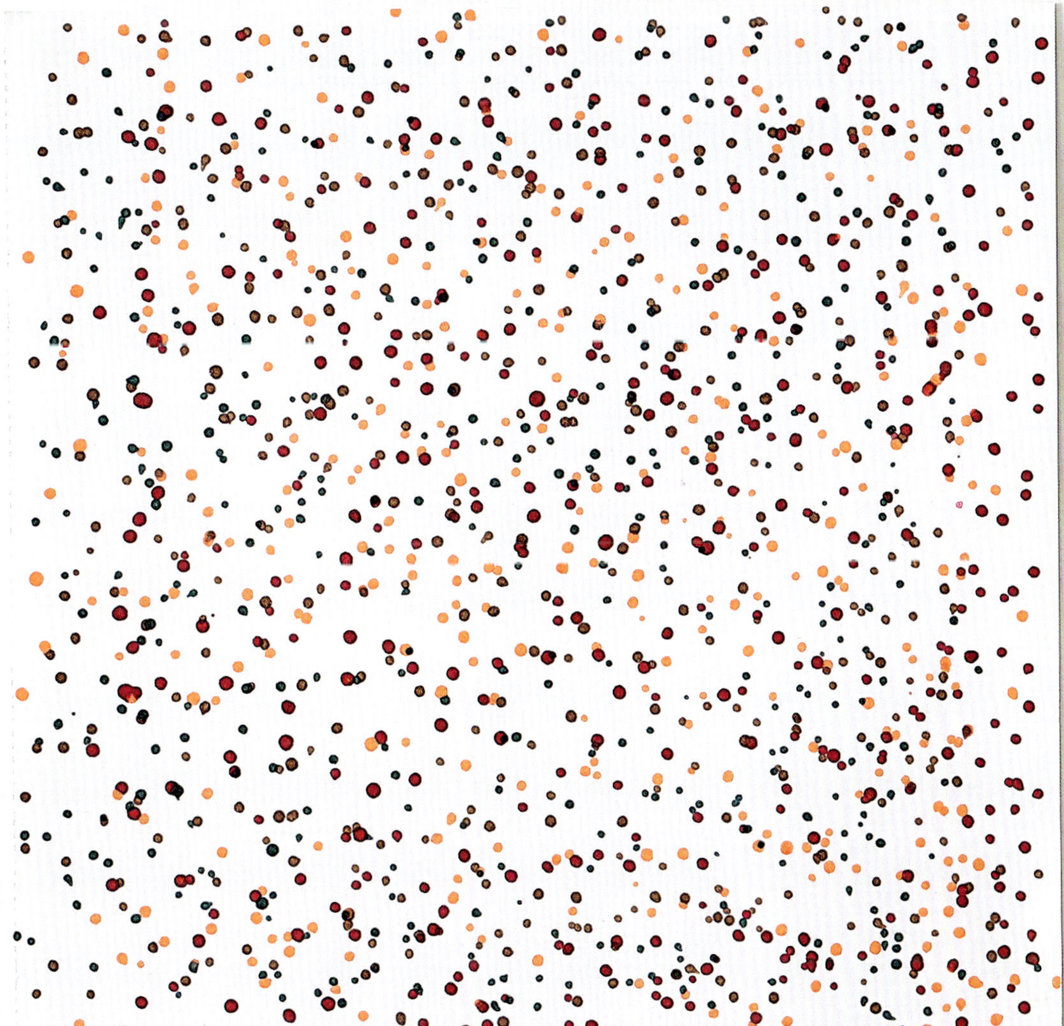

EXERCISE 20

Puddles of imperfection

Working with uncontrolled paint flow teaches acceptance and surrender. Instead of forcing order, you allow beauty to emerge in a soft and unpredictable way.

INSTRUCTIONS

1. Mix the paint with enough water or pouring medium to achieve a pouring consistency.
2. Pour or drip the paint onto your canvas or board. Let it spread and mix naturally.
3. Tilt the canvas or board to encourage flow, or gently guide the paint by moving it around with a spatula or your fingers.
4. Let the piece dry fully. Come back later to see the outcome.

WHAT YOU NEED

- ⇛ Canvas or board
- ⇛ Acrylic paint
- ⇛ Pouring medium (optional)
- ⇛ Cup or container
- ⇛ Spatula (optional)

THERAPIST'S INSIGHT

Life is unpredictable, and this can be difficult for an anxious brain. By practising ways to cope with change and respond to chaos, we can reduce discomfort around the unknown.

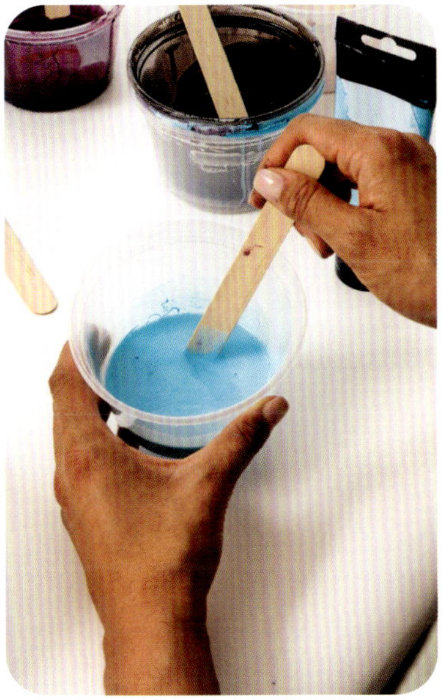

Step 1

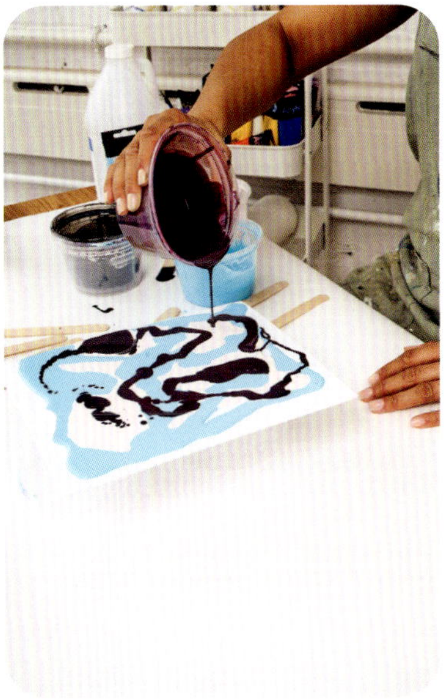

Step 2

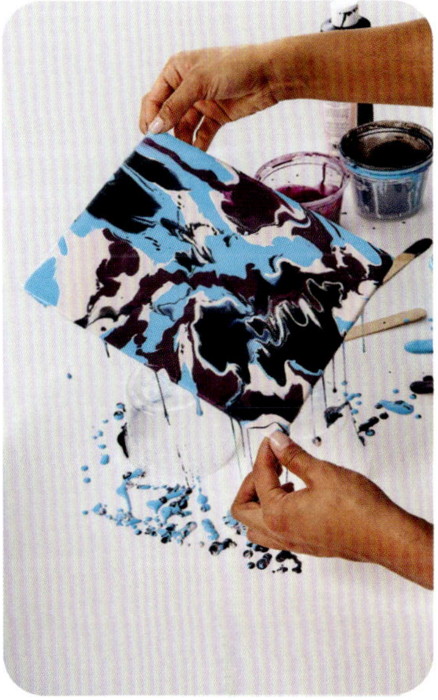

Step 3

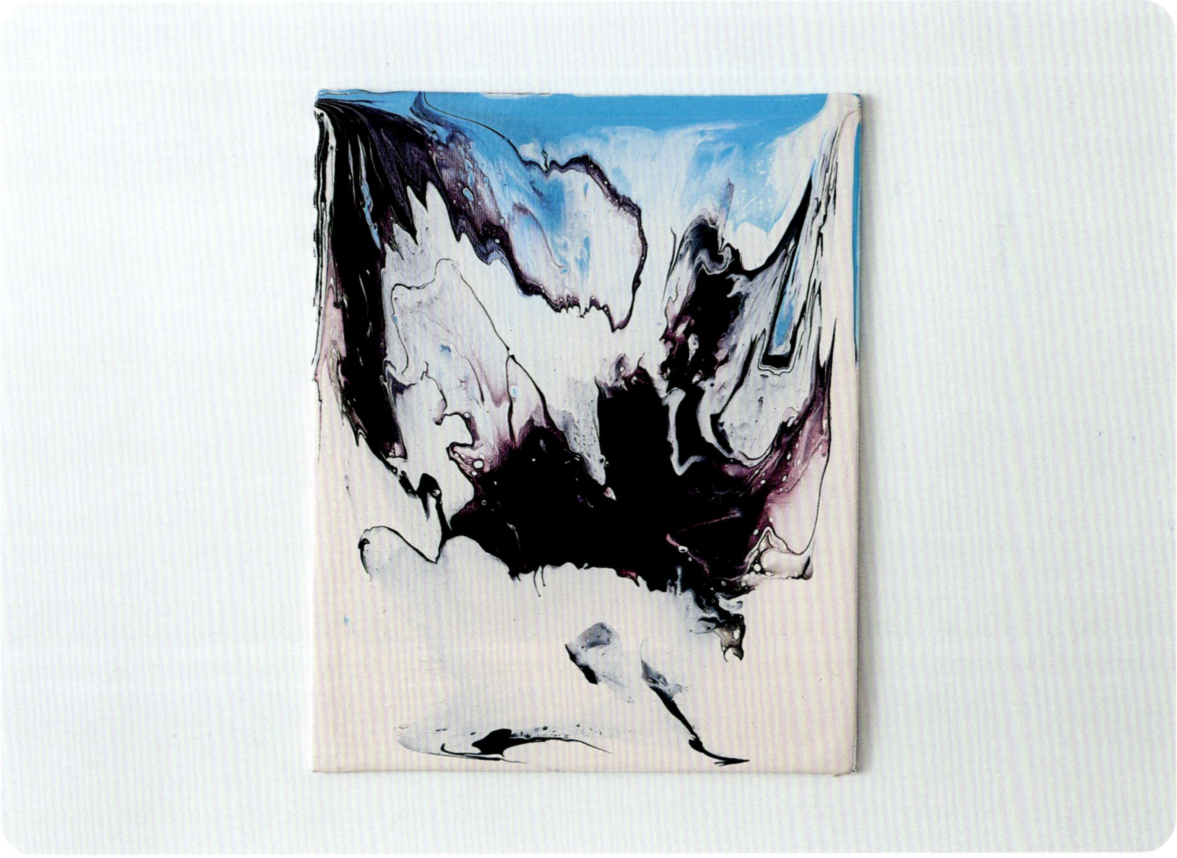

CHAPTER 3

EMBRACING UNCERTAINTY

Introduction

Uncertainty can feel especially uncomfortable for neurodivergent minds. Not knowing what comes next, how something will turn out, or whether you're 'doing it right' can trigger anxiety, self-doubt or a need to control. Yet uncertainty is also where creativity begins.

Art can be a gentle practice in letting go. The exercises in this chapter invite you to release planning, prediction and perfection and instead notice and respond to what happens in each moment. I encourage you to meet uncertainty with curiosity. There is no 'wrong' outcome here. Each page becomes a record of your willingness to stay present even when the path is unclear. For many neurodivergent people, this can be deeply freeing. It allows creativity to exist without pressure, rules or comparison. It also builds trust – both in the process and in yourself.

As you move through this chapter, notice how your body responds when you do not know what is coming next. Do you tense, rush, pause or resist? See if you can soften into that moment instead, allowing the artwork to unfold without needing to control it. Embracing uncertainty means moving forwards even without having all the answers – one line, one shape, one breath at a time.

THERAPIST'S NOTE

Accepting uncertainty helps promote emotional resilience. When outcomes are unclear, the brain interprets this as a threat, even when no immediate danger is present. Life, relationships and experiences are never predictable, and learning to accept this can help us move through the discomfort with greater ease, reducing the intensity of unexpected moments. The exercises in this chapter will help you to reframe your thoughts, including somatic practices to help calm the nervous system.

EXERCISE 21

Blindfold art

Drawing without looking helps you to let go of control and expectations. It invites curiosity and trust in the process. This helps quiet perfectionism and allows creative flow to lead instead of logic.

INSTRUCTIONS

1. Place your chosen materials in front of you then blindfold yourself, or close your eyes.
2. Get comfortable and make sure everything is within easy reach (have someone with you to guide you if that makes you feel more at ease).
3. Begin drawing or painting freely using your chosen tools. Alternatively, use just your hands for a more sensory experience.
4. Stop painting whenever you feel ready to.
5. Open your eyes and see your creation.

WHAT YOU NEED

⇛ Paper or canvas

⇛ Your favourite tools and materials

⇛ Blindfold (or simply close your eyes)

TIP

Choose colours that bring you joy.

THERAPIST'S INSIGHT

When one sense is restricted, the others become more aware. Touch activates the parasympathetic nervous system – the 'rest and digest' state – lowering cortisol levels, reducing stress and creating a sense of safety. This can calm you down and help you connect to your creative side.

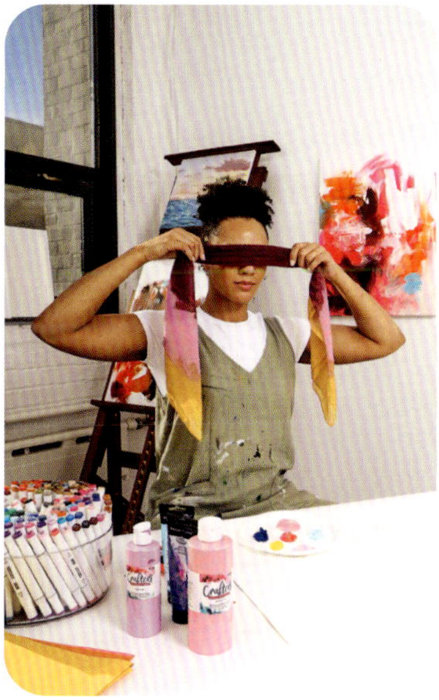

Step 1

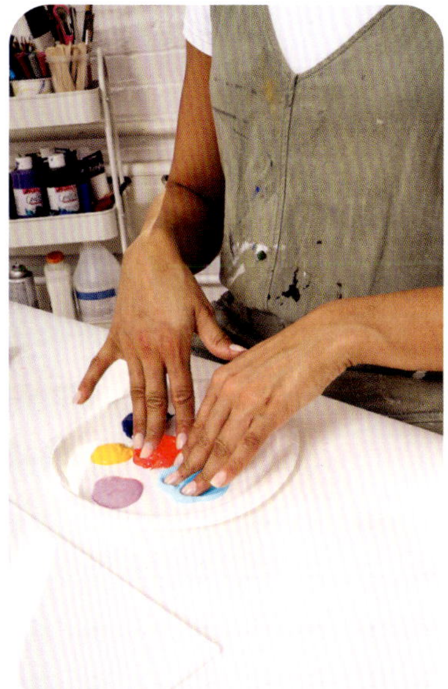

Step 2

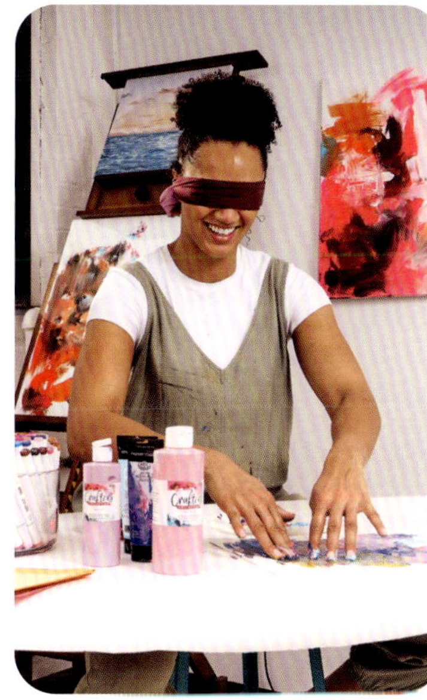

Step 3

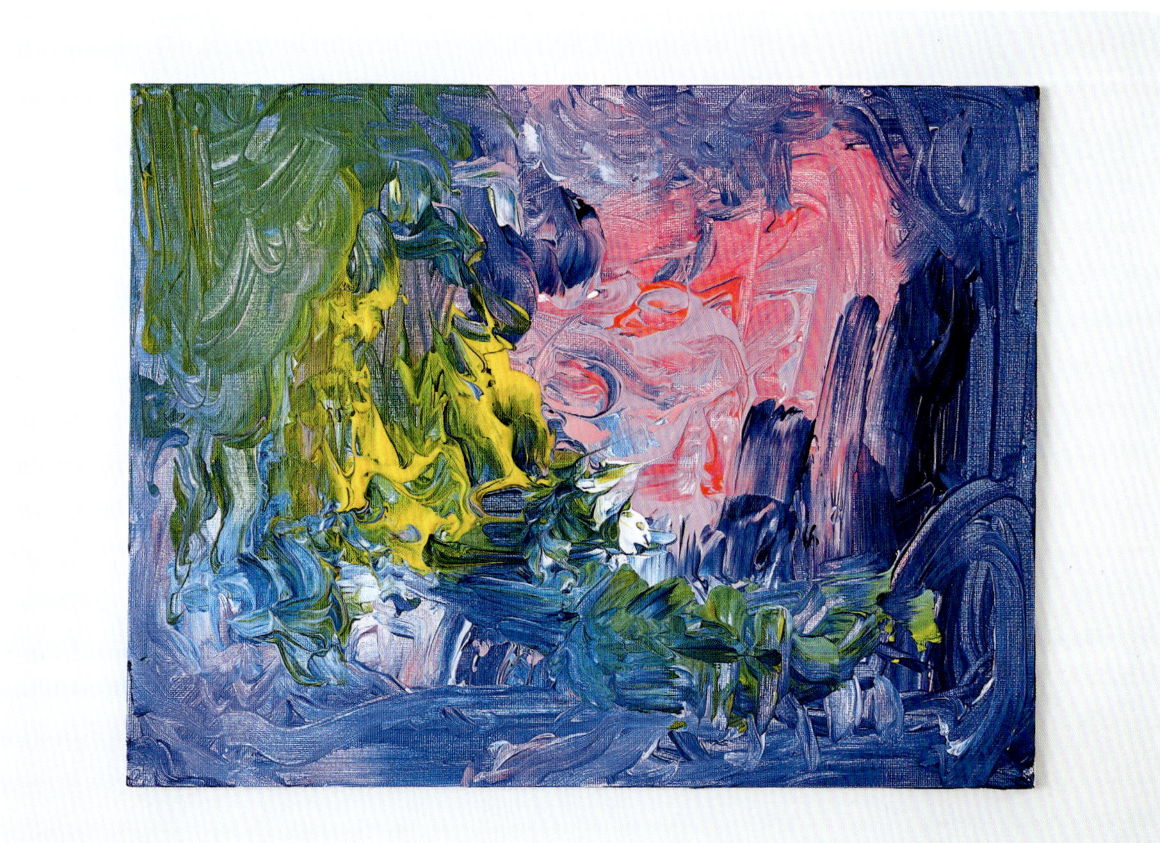

EXERCISE 22

Swap hands drawing

Using your non-dominant hand can help quiet the analytical brain and activate new neural pathways. It can make space for imperfection and reconnect art with play.

INSTRUCTIONS

1. Hold your drawing tool of choice in your non-dominant hand.
2. Choose a simple subject, or draw abstractly.
3. Move slowly as you draw and notice how it feels to release control.
4. Keep going even if it feels awkward or messy.
5. Let the strangeness be part of the process.

WHAT YOU NEED

⇛ Paper

⇛ Any drawing tool of choice, such as paint and brush, pencil, pen or markers

THERAPIST'S INSIGHT

Drawing in this way encourages you to slow down because it requires more thought and patience. By moving your hand more consciously, you can increase feelings of safety and foster creativity.

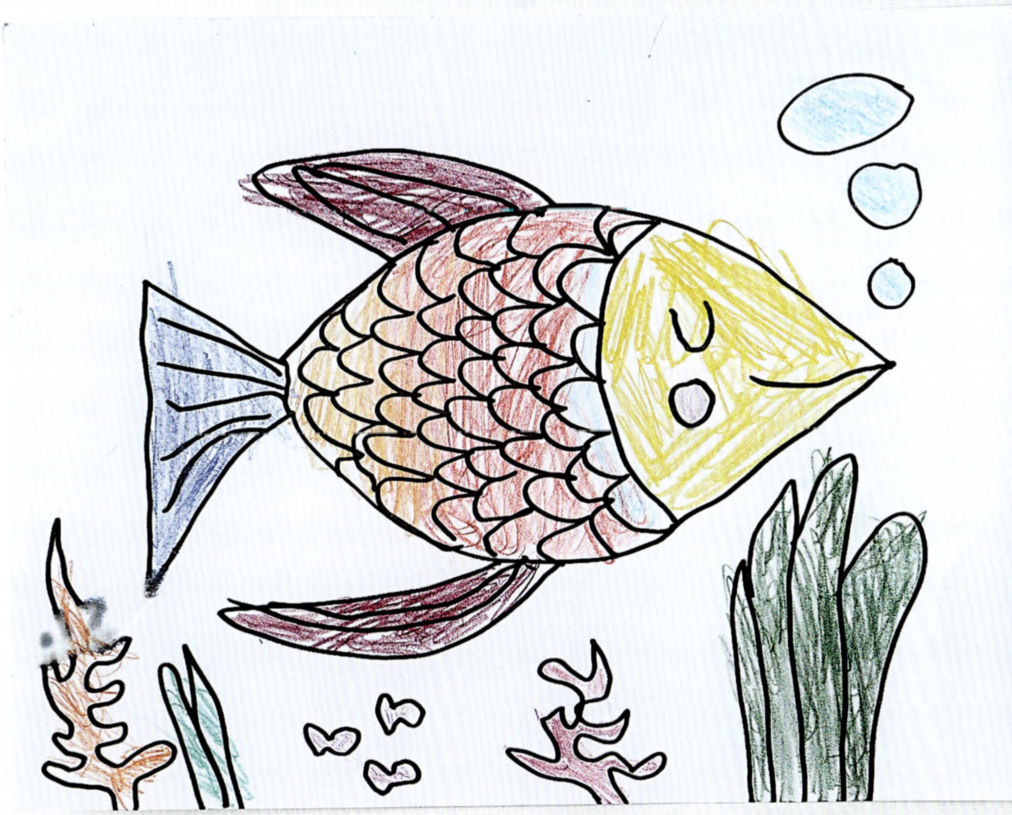

EXERCISE 23

The pebble exercise

As the pebble moves unpredictably across the page, it shows how beauty can appear when you have surrendered control. It mirrors life's flow and encourages a sense of peace in not knowing the outcome.

INSTRUCTIONS

1. Place the pebble on your paper.
2. Hold your pen, pencil or pastel lightly against it.
3. Begin guiding the pebble with your hand, letting the pen trace its movement.
4. Move slowly – don't force the direction.
5. When finished, observe the organic paths you have created.

WHAT YOU NEED

⇛ Paper

⇛ Pen, pencil or soft pastels

⇛ Small pebble or smooth stone

THERAPIST'S INSIGHT

Focusing in this way keeps your attention in the present, quietening overthinking. This supports oxytocin release and lowers cortisol, the stress hormone, helping your brain feel safer and steadier.

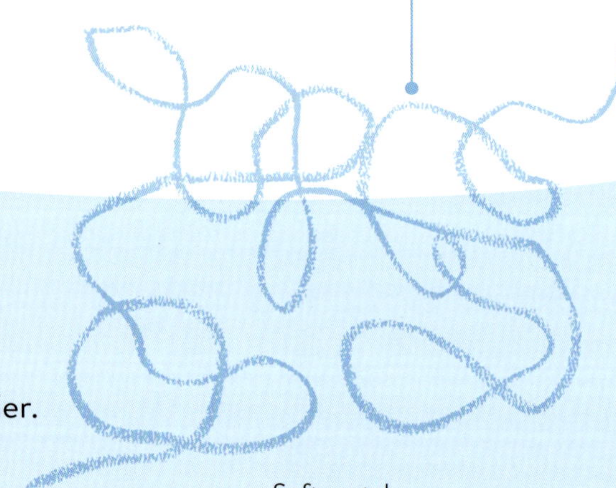

Soft pastel

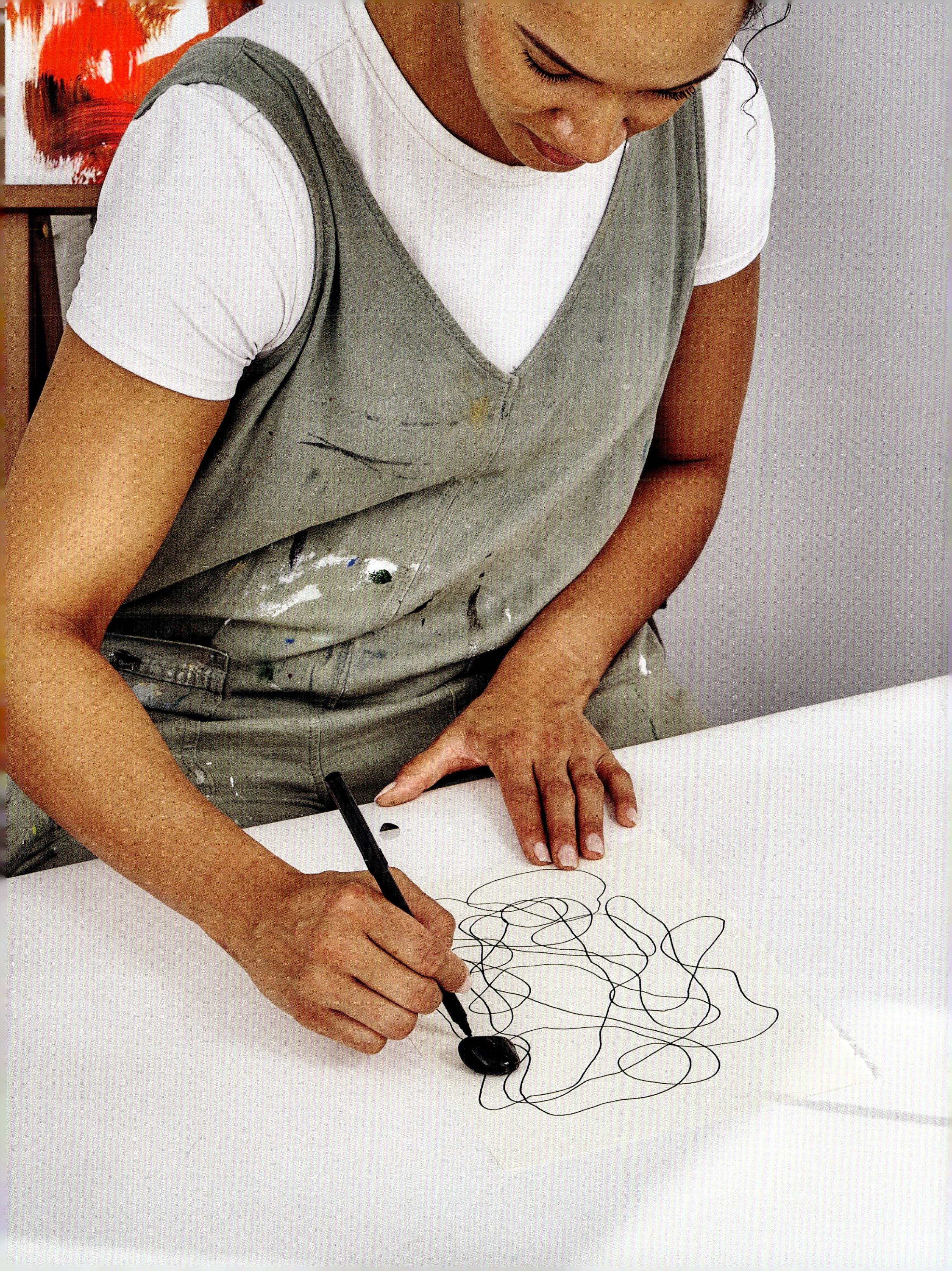

EXERCISE 24

Chance colours

Letting chance make colour choices removes the need to make decisions. This gives the neurodivergent brain more freedom and reduces overwhelm.

INSTRUCTIONS

1. Randomly pick three colours, without looking.
2. Use only those colours on your paper and use them freely.
3. Allow the colours to mix, overlap or clash without judgement.
4. Focus on movement, not perfection.
5. Stop when what you have done feels balanced enough for you.

WHAT YOU NEED

- ⇛ Paper
- ⇛ A selection of paints and brushes, markers or pencils

THERAPIST'S INSIGHT

This exercise reflects a core idea from Acceptance and Commitment Therapy (ACT): noticing and accepting whatever arrives. Just as you may hope for one colour but pick another, ACT encourages flexibility in facing unexpected thoughts, feelings or experiences.

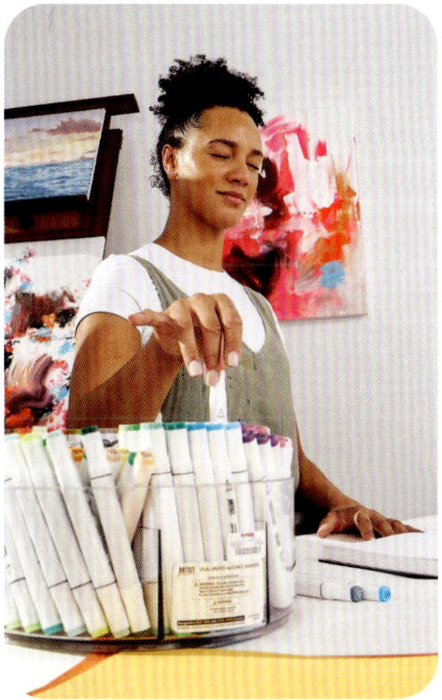

Step 1

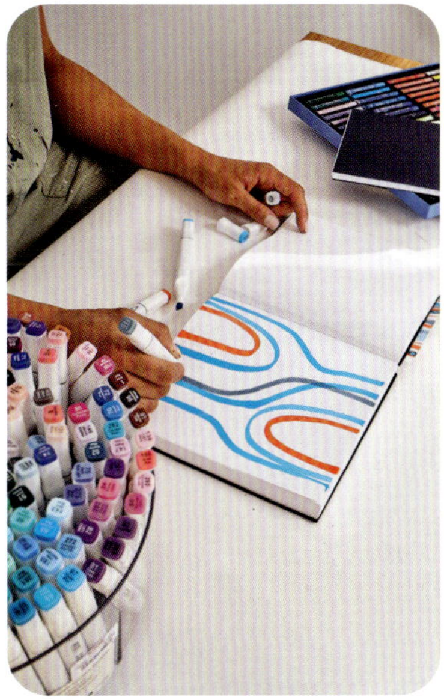

Step 2

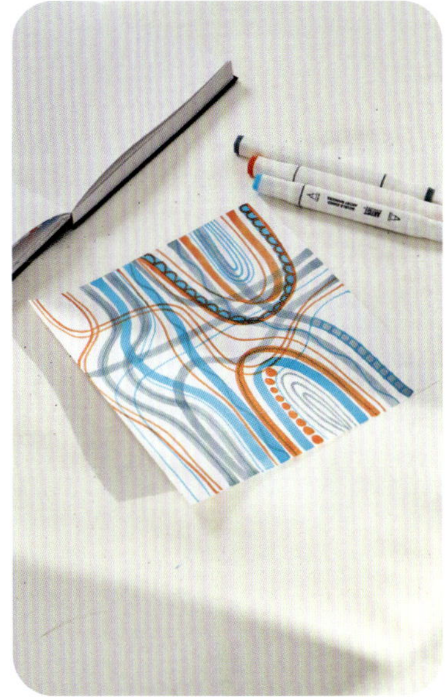

Step 5

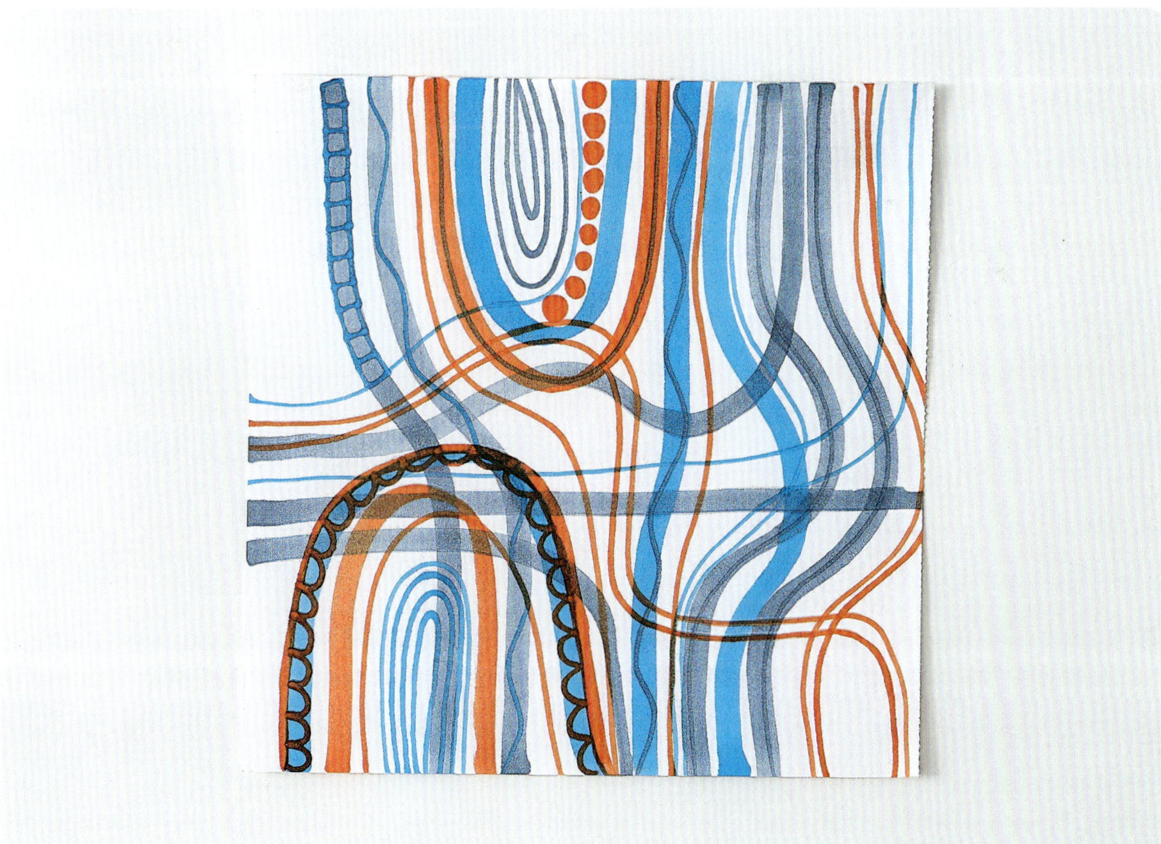

EXERCISE 25

Ink bloom experiment

Adding an element of randomness turns pressure into play. It teaches flexibility and curiosity, rather than rigid control.

INSTRUCTIONS

1. Drop a tiny bit of ink or very watery paint onto the paper.
2. Blow gently through a straw to spread the ink.
3. Let the ink 'bloom' form branching shapes.
4. When the ink is dry, add delicate pen lines responding to the shapes.
5. Repeat steps 1–4, if you like, adding more ink then more pen lines, building the image gradually until it feels right to you.

WHAT YOU NEED

- Paper
- Ink or watery paint
- Straw
- Fineliner or marker

AFFIRMATION

I allow life to surprise me.

THERAPIST'S INSIGHT

This exercise helps you cope with uncertainty as you cannot control how the ink moves. Blowing through the straw with slow, steady breaths triggers the parasympathetic nervous system, slows your heart rate and reduces stress.

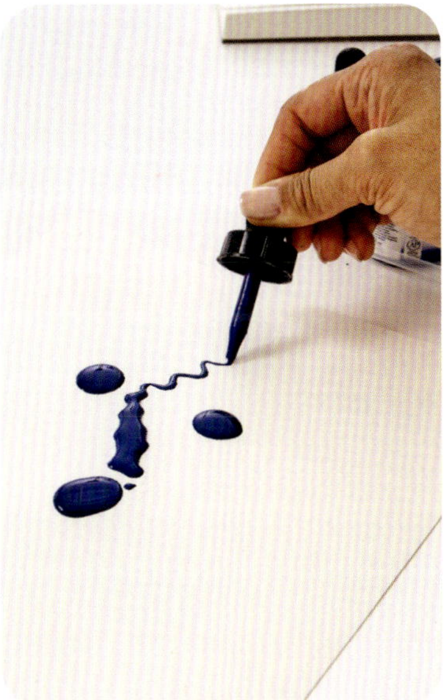

Step 1

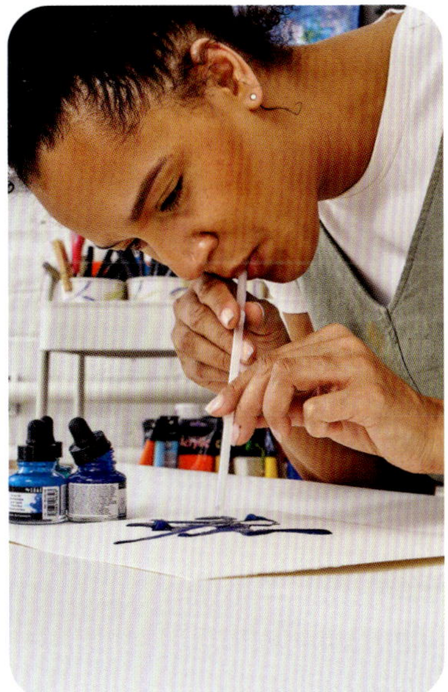

Step 2

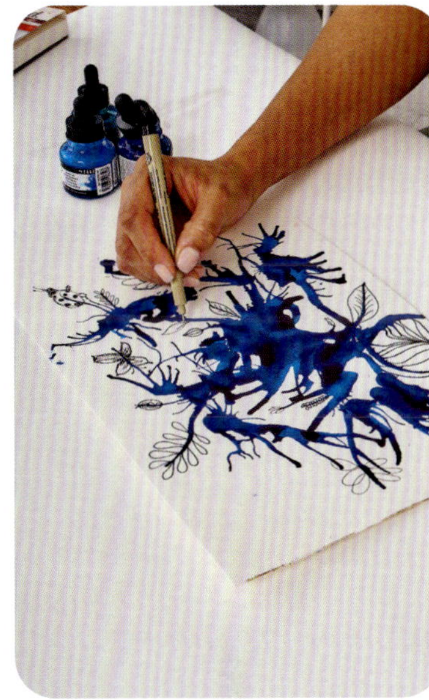

Step 4

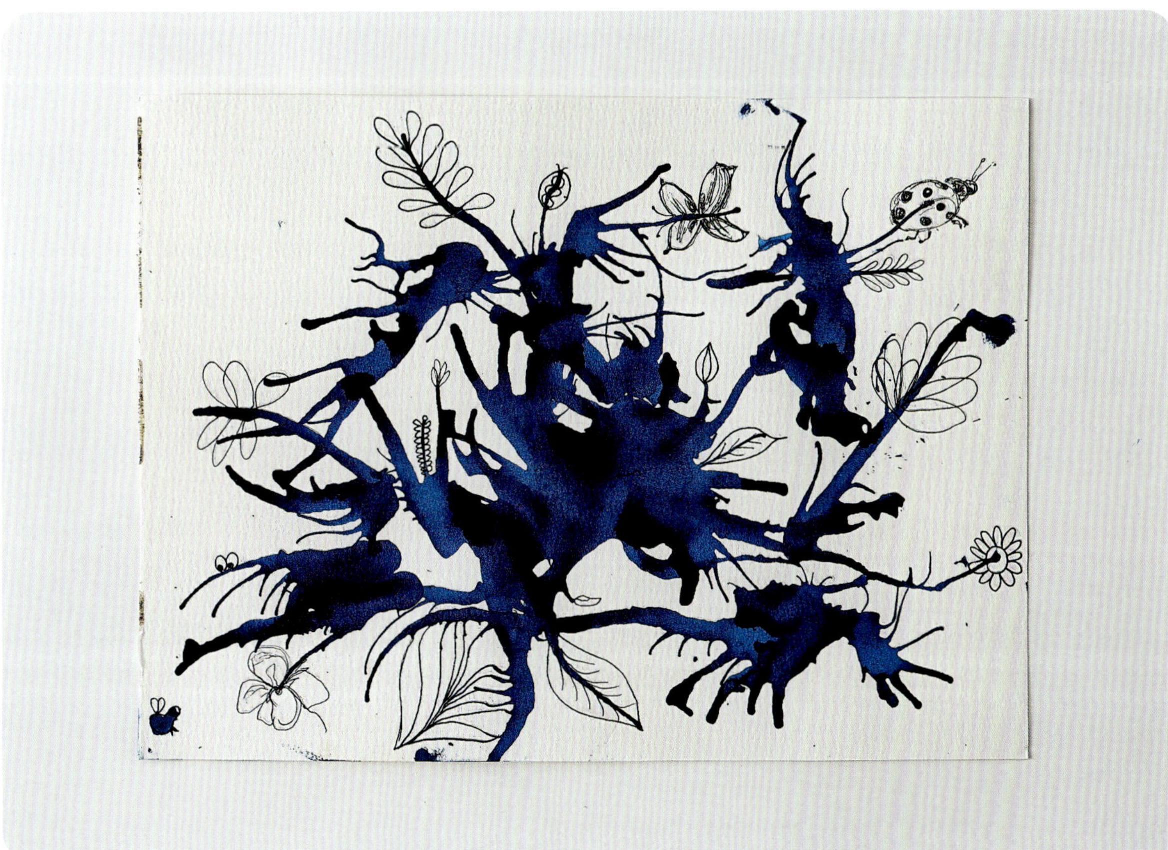

EXERCISE 26

Follow the music

Responding to sound through movement connects body and emotion. It encourages instinctive expression rather than mental control. It reduces anxiety and promotes a natural flow.

INSTRUCTIONS

1. Play a song that moves you.
2. Close your eyes or soften your gaze. Really feel the music.
3. Hold your art tool of choice and respond intuitively to the music, letting your hand move with the rhythm – fast or slow, light or heavy.
4. Do not plan or judge the marks.
5. When the music stops, take a deep breath and observe what you have created.

WHAT YOU NEED

⇒ Paper

⇒ Art tool of choice, such as oil pastel or paint and brush

⇒ Music of choice

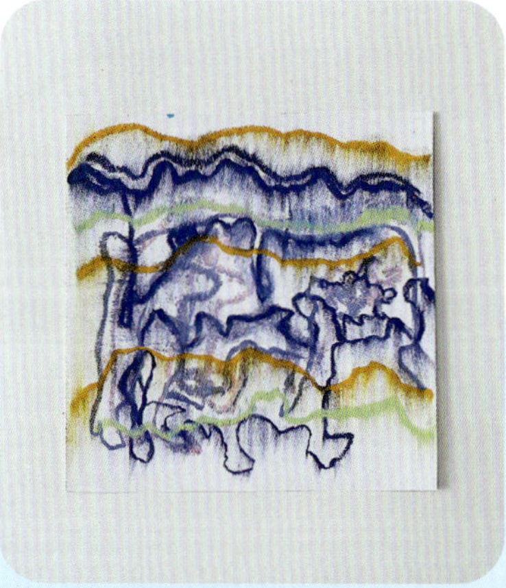

Alternative drawing

THERAPIST'S INSIGHT

Moving your brush or pen in response to music helps you engage with your body. Somatic movement helps regulate the nervous system by fostering a deep mind-body connection, creating a sense of safety and calm.

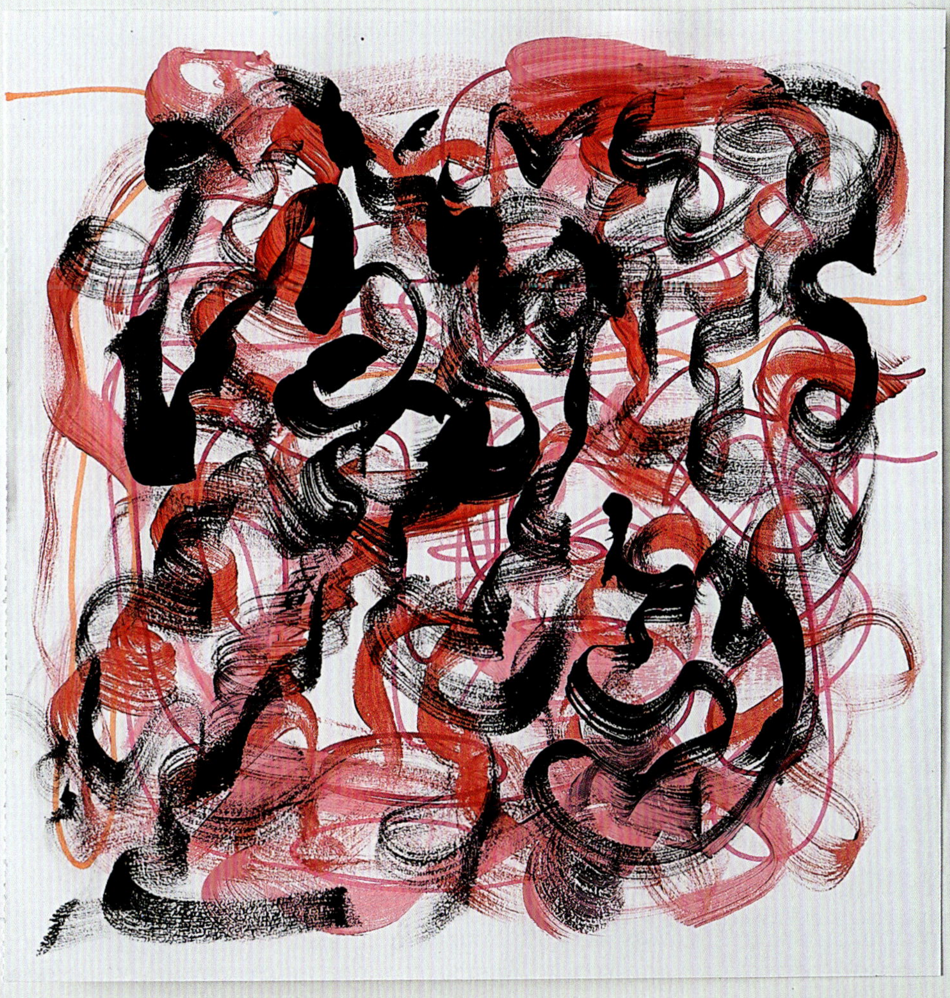

EXERCISE 27

Surface & surrender

This exercise invites you to work with an uneven surface that cannot be fully controlled.

When we introduce sand or textured material into the painting process, the artwork responds in unexpected ways. Lines break, paint catches, marks skip. Yet unpredictability doesn't mean failure – it simply means responding instead of forcing. For neurodivergent creatives, this helps loosen perfectionism and control, while building trust in adaptability and presence.

WHAT YOU NEED

- Paper, card or canvas (thicker surfaces work best)
- Palette knife or old card
- Small container
- Textured material, such as sand, soil, salt, crushed shells, grit or similar
- PVA glue
- Acrylic paint (optional)
- Gloves (if using glue)
- Metallic pen, or paint for later detailing (optional)
- Gold leaf (optional)

INSTRUCTIONS

1. In a small container, combine your textured material with glue. You can add a little paint if you like, or leave it neutral.
2. Using a palette knife or old card, spread the mixture onto the surface of the paper, card or canvas. Let it be imperfect.

THERAPIST'S INSIGHT

Sensory overload is often experienced by neurodivergent brains. This exercise helps you redirect sensory overload into organized chaos while reducing the need to mask emotions in order to fit in or manage social situations.

3. Play with the composition by moving the mixture around.
4. Add more paint in places, and sprinkle extra texture where it feels right.
5. Pause and notice: take a moment to feel the surface visually and physically. Notice how it's forming without you fully controlling it.
6. Allow the piece to dry fully. This pause is part of the practice.
7. Once dry, add gentle details, if you like – such as lines, colour or gold leaf – responding to the texture rather than covering it.

SENSORY CUE

Notice the resistance beneath your hands. Let the surface decide where the textured material settles.

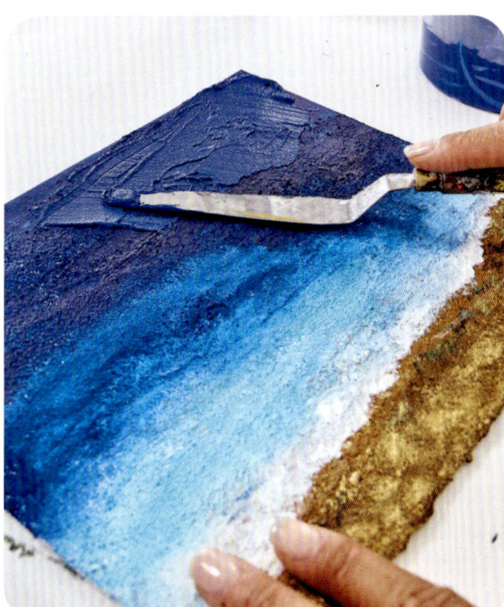

Step 3

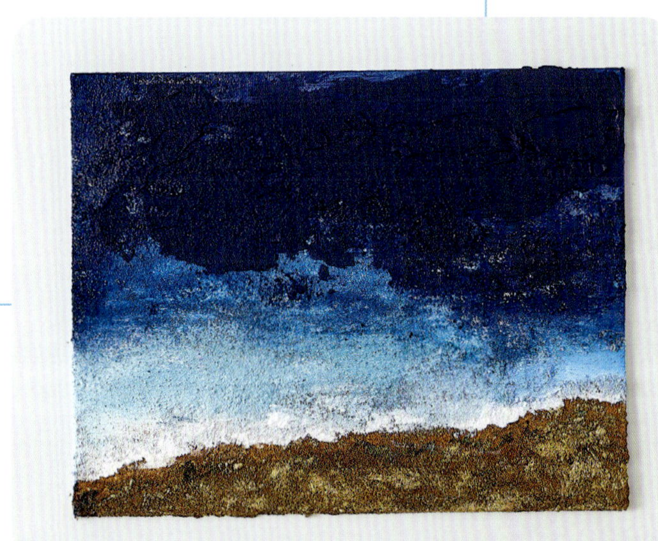

EXERCISE 28

Spill & respond

Accidental marks often spark the imagination. Learning to respond to them rather than control them fosters adaptability and resilience.

INSTRUCTIONS

1. Gently spill or drop the coffee or tea onto your paper. You can tilt the page slightly to let the liquid move and spread naturally.
2. Pause and watch the shapes that form. Try not to control or judge them – just notice.
3. Allow the paper to dry completely. Once it is dry, look for forms, patterns or images within the stains.
4. Using your chosen art materials, slowly add lines, details or colour to bring those shapes to life. Let your imagination guide you – there is no right or wrong outcome.

WHAT YOU NEED

- ⇛ Paper (the thicker the better)
- ⇛ Leftover coffee or tea, cooled
- ⇛ Your favourite art materials – anything you enjoy using

THERAPIST'S INSIGHT

This exercise focuses on the process, not the outcome, an approach is used in Cognitive Behavioural Therapy (CBT), which connects thought patterns, feelings and behaviour to break cycles of negative thinking. By responding differently to spilling paint, you train your brain to be calmer and more positive when negative emotions are triggered.

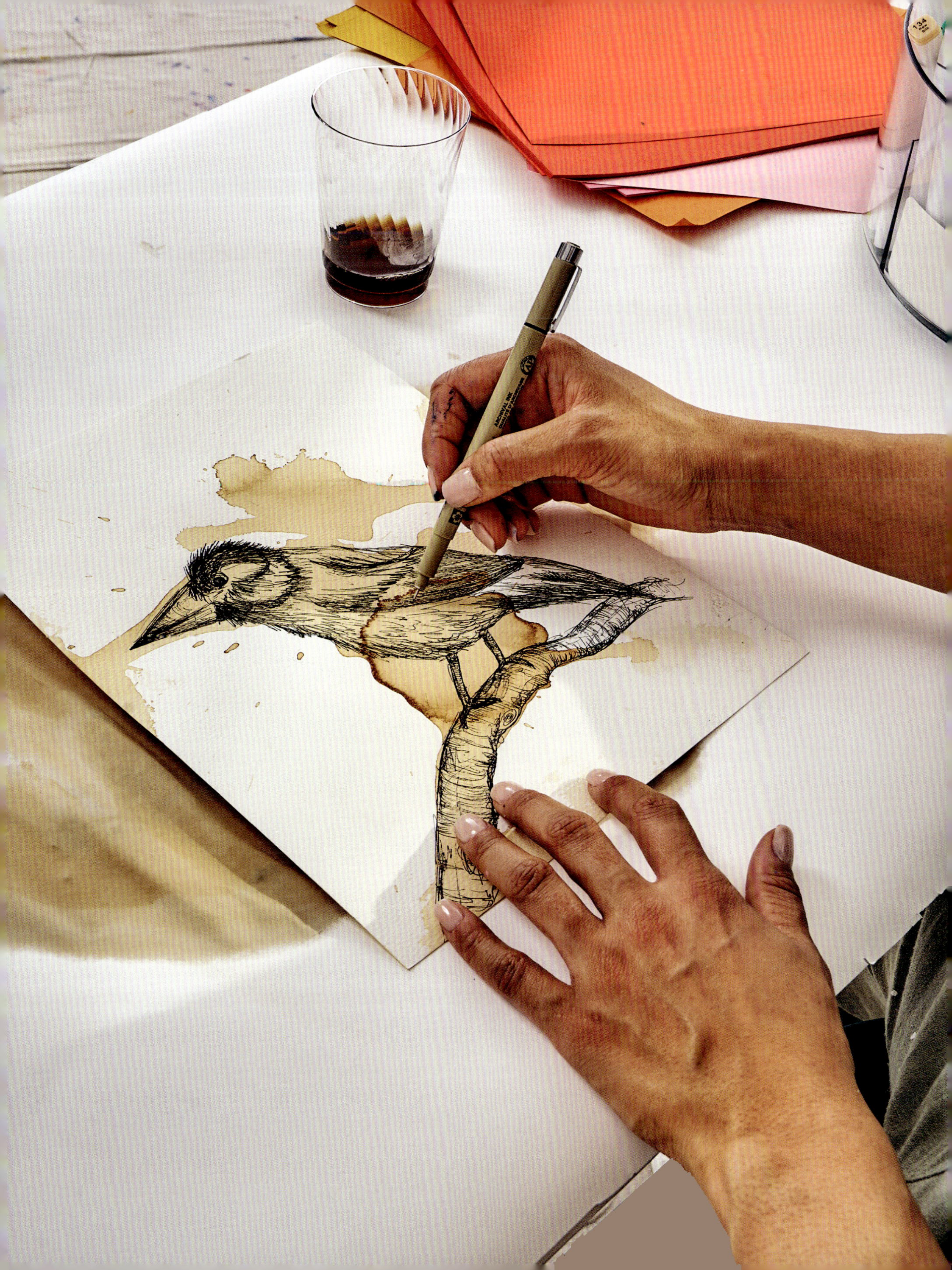

EXERCISE 29

Chaos to composition

Transforming randomness into a gentle structure reminds us that we can bring order to inner chaos without erasing its energy. This builds creative confidence and calm.

INSTRUCTIONS

1. Fill the page with random marks, splats or lines.
2. Pause and look at what stands out.
3. Choose a few areas to emphasize with patterns or colours.
4. Gently connect or balance elements across the page.
5. Let harmony emerge slowly from the randomness on the page.

WHAT YOU NEED

- ⇛ Paper
- ⇛ Paint and brush
- ⇛ Pen

THERAPIST'S INSIGHT

Creating random marks can release tension. Pausing after helps you regain control. This process strengthens brain connections and builds resilience, showing that a calm response helps you handle whatever arises.

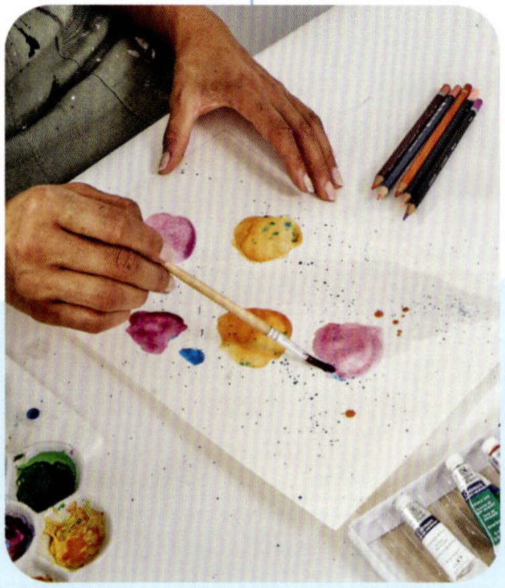

Step 1

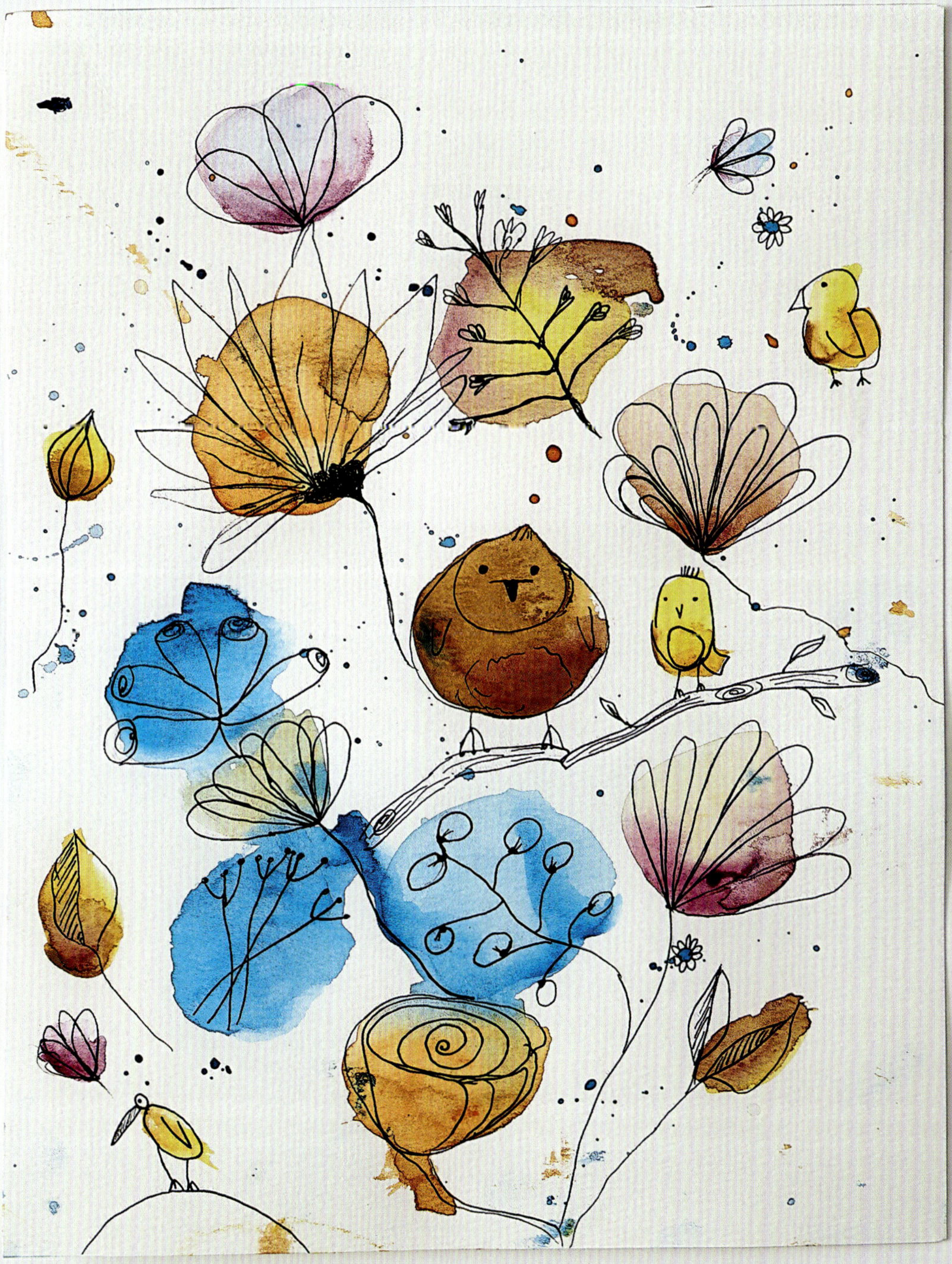

EXERCISE 30

The pebble mandala

This exercise uses mandala art therapy, but combines it with the strong focus-on-now emphasis of the pebble exercise on page 70. The result is a balanced combination of structure and chaos.

INSTRUCTIONS

1. Place your pebble in the centre of the page.
2. Let it lead your pen in circular, spiralling or wandering lines.
3. Then build tiny repeating patterns between the lines – dots, petals, arcs and shapes.
4. Each repetition becomes grounding and meditative.
5. Colour the spaces created where the lines overlap. Use colours that make you feel calm.

WHAT YOU NEED

- ⇒ Paper
- ⇒ Pebble
- ⇒ Pen
- ⇒ Colour pens or pencils

THERAPIST'S INSIGHT

The meditative drawing inside the shapes created by the pebble brings back order, calm and mindfulness and helps to reduce anxiety.

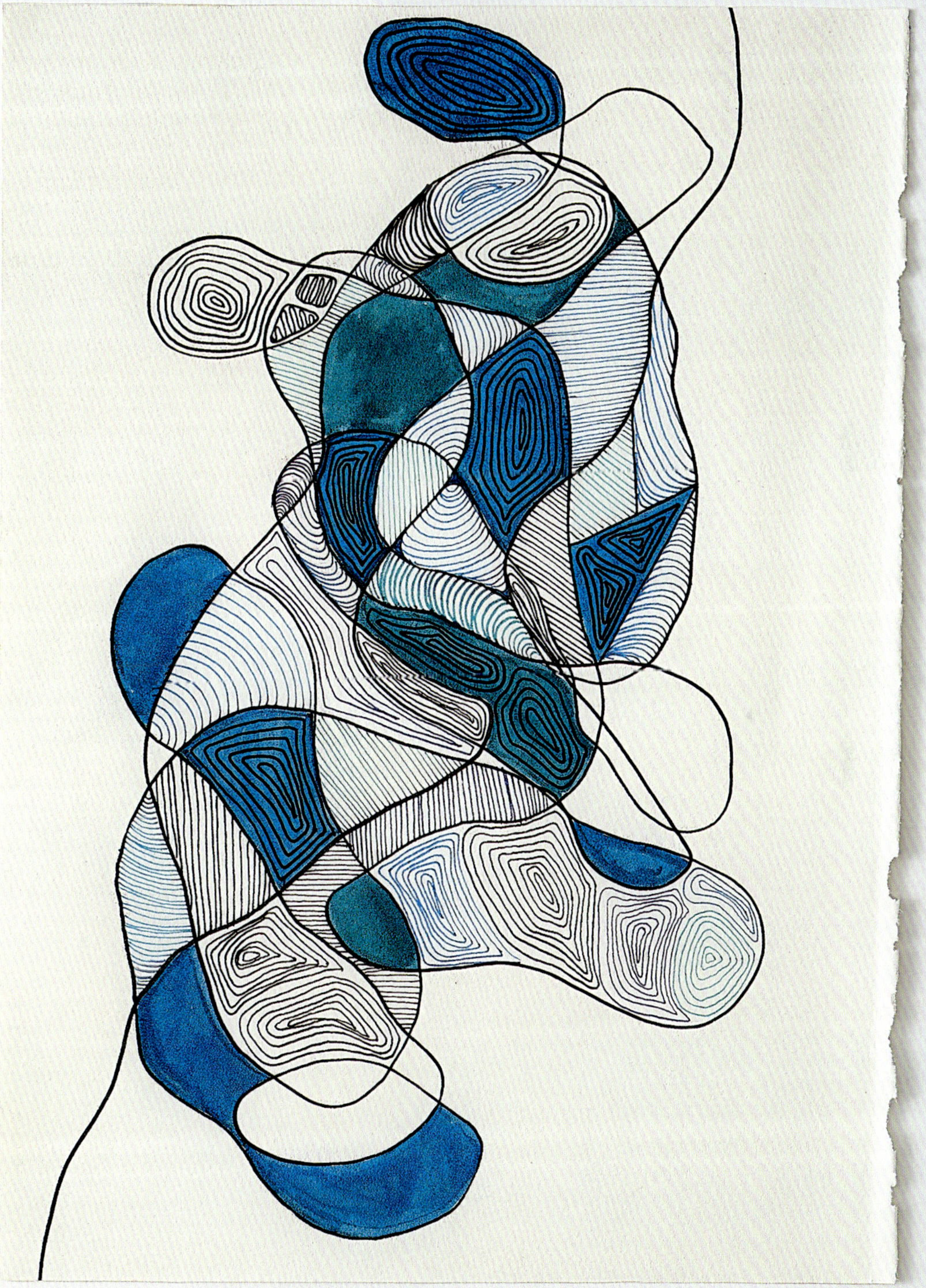

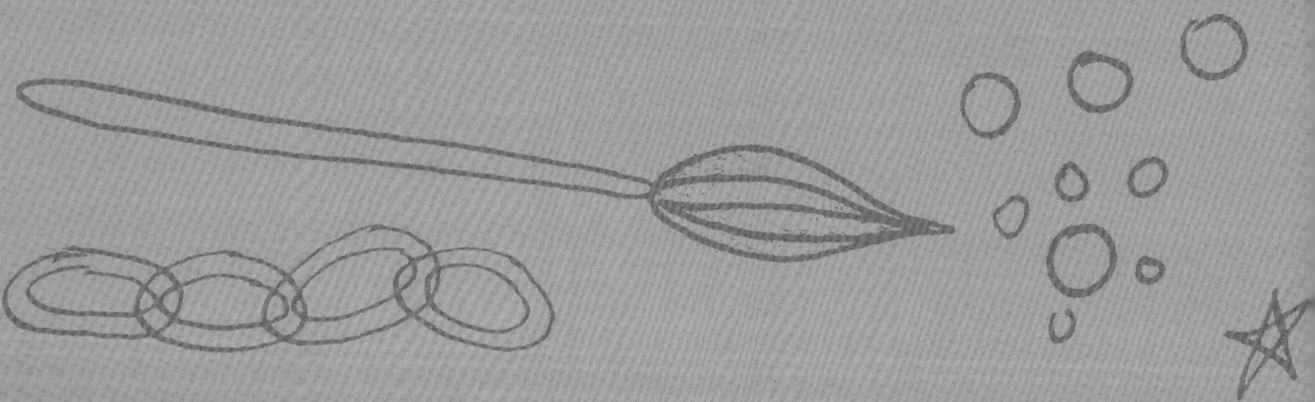

CHAPTER 4

NEURO-DIVERGENT STRENGTHS

Introduction

So much of neurodivergent life is spent adapting, masking or trying to fit into systems that were not designed for you. Over time this can make creativity feel pressured, too full of effort or tied to self-judgement.

This chapter is an invitation to gently shift perspective. Rather than focusing on what feels difficult, the exercises here are designed to highlight what already works – the strengths that often come with neurodivergent minds. Sensory awareness. Pattern recognition. Emotional depth. Intuition. The ability to notice what others might overlook.

The practices here encourage you to work with your natural rhythms rather than against them. You'll be invited to break things into smaller parts, respond to sensation instead of expectation, and let the body guide the creative process. For many people, this can reduce overwhelm and make creativity feel more accessible and enjoyable.

You do not need to complete every exercise or move through them in order. This chapter is about choice, permission and trusting yourself. It is not asking you to change how your mind works. It is inviting you to recognize the quiet strengths that were there all along.

THERAPIST'S NOTE

Many neurodivergent individuals learn to adapt, mask or suppress parts of themselves so they can fit into social situations. But those of us with differently wired brains also have marked strengths which are often overlooked. These include deep focus, noticing patterns, problem-solving, innovation and exceptional creativity. It's hugely important to remind ourselves of these positive strengths, and this affirming chapter helps you reflect on these. Shifting from worrying about your differences to working with your strengths helps you embrace all parts of yourself and celebrate who you are.

EXERCISE 31

Trace the overwhelm

Repetition provides regulation and focus. Creating patterns by hand can feel like 'stimming on paper', giving both comfort and release while celebrating your rhythmic, intuitive mind.

INSTRUCTIONS

1. Begin by drawing or painting small repeated marks – circles, waves, lines or dots.
2. Let the shapes grow across the page freely.
3. Follow your hand's rhythm – fast or slow, detailed or loose.
4. If it feels comfortable, you can close your eyes and keep drawing, letting your hand follow the movement and pattern you have already started.
5. Add more colours if you like.

WHAT YOU NEED

⇛ Paper

⇛ Your favourite art materials – anything you enjoy using

AFFIRMATION

My patterns are power – not perfection.

THERAPIST'S INSIGHT

Some neurodivergent brains look for extra sensory stimulation to feel calm and balanced. The repetition in this exercise helps release built-up energy in the body. It also supports sensory regulation, helps improve focus and can reduce feelings of anxiety.

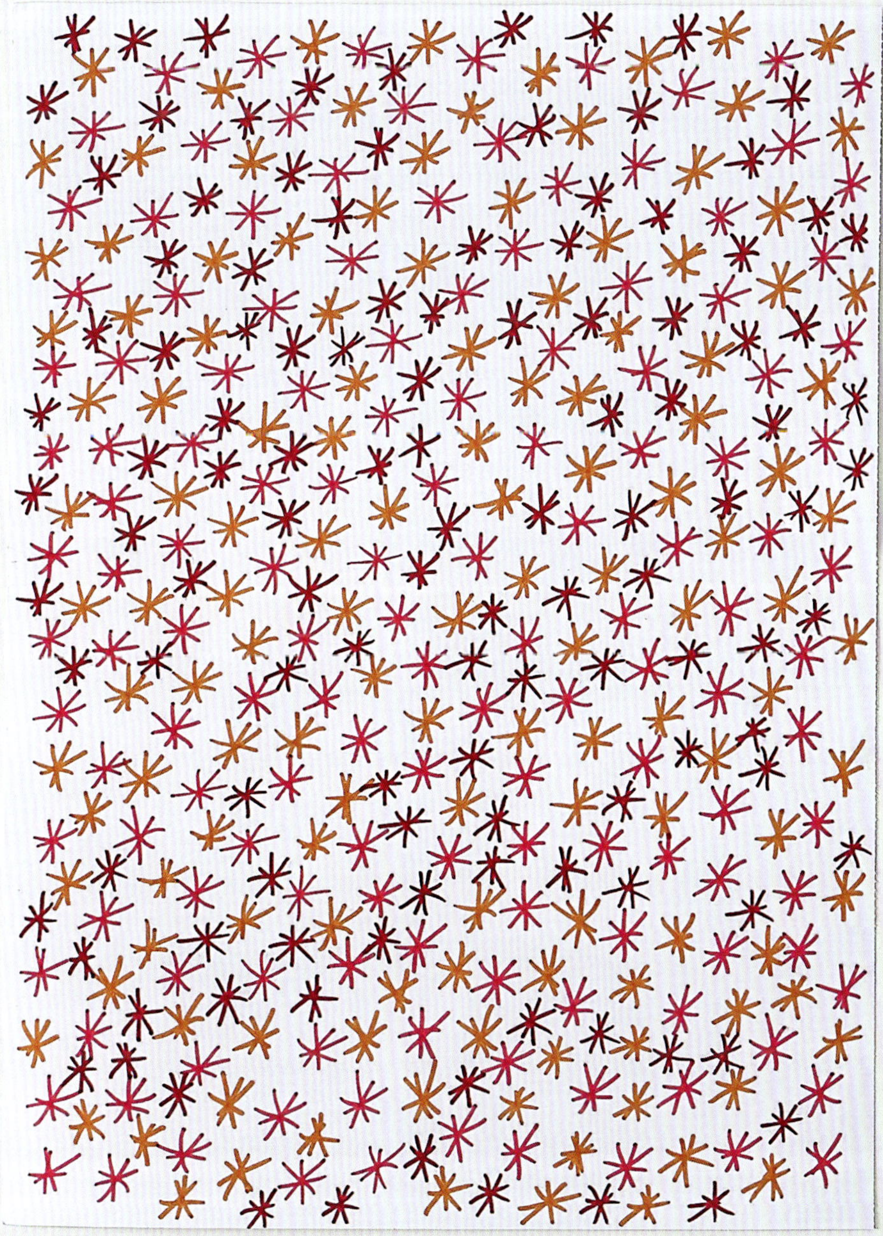

EXERCISE 32

The quiet space

Drawing or imagining a 'safe space' allows you to externalize calm and belonging. It strengthens emotional safety and helps ground you after sensory overload.

INSTRUCTIONS

1. Close your eyes and imagine a space that feels peaceful and safe.
2. On paper, begin drawing or painting that space – real or imagined.
3. Add comforting symbols – light, plants, blankets or abstract forms.
4. Fill the space with calming textures, shapes or colours.
5. Let the page hold that peace for you.

WHAT YOU NEED

⇒ Paper

⇒ Pencils, markers or paint and brush

THERAPIST'S INSIGHT

This exercise guides the brain to create a plan for a peaceful, unthreatening place. It helps people think through what a realistic safe space could look like so it can be drawn on when needed.

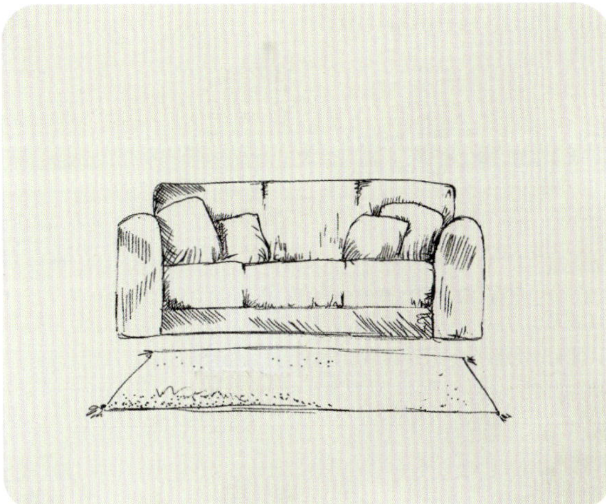

Step 2

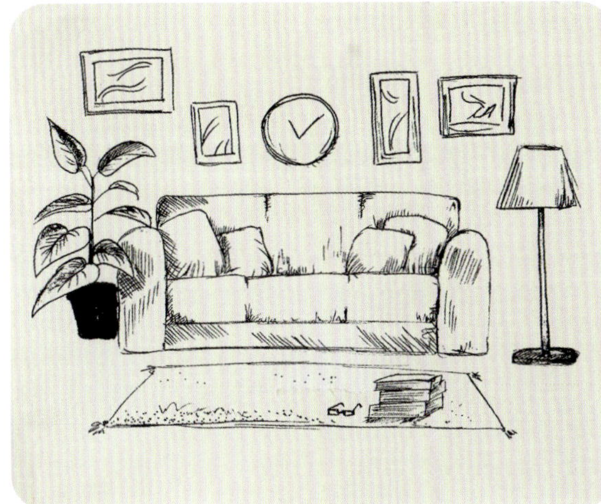

Step 3

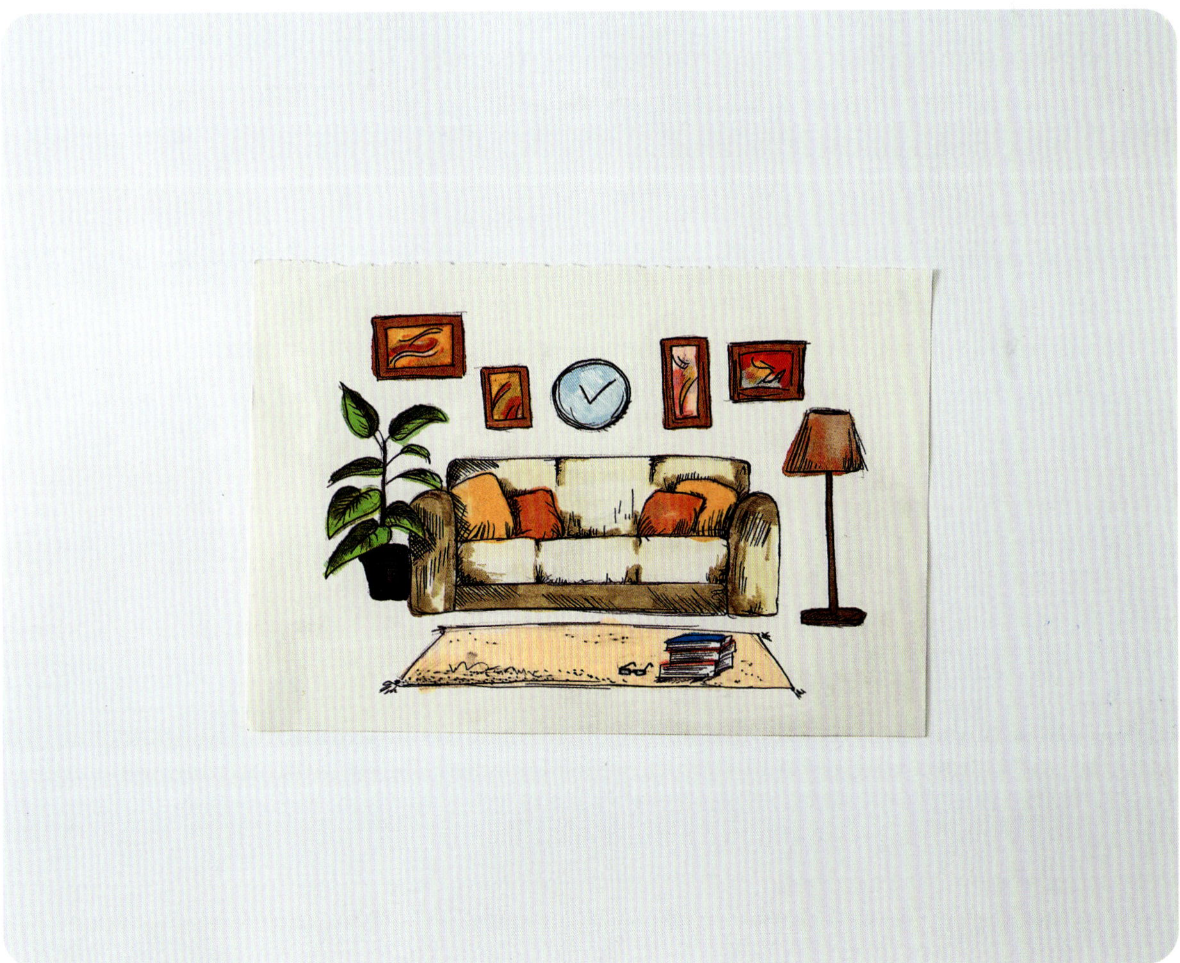

EXERCISE 33

Strength self-portrait

Using symbols and colours to show who you are builds self-esteem. It celebrates your creativity, your intuition and the way you understand the world.

INSTRUCTIONS

1. Think of qualities you love or admire in yourself, such as kindness, resilience and curiosity, then choose whether you would like to make a figurative or an abstract portrait.
2. Assign colours to your strengths – for example red for passion and yellow for kindness – and draw using these colours. Alternatively, you can position shapes to represent your strengths in a more abstract way. For example, you could roll paper into spirals and glue them to the surface.
3. Add lines or textures that feel like 'you'.
4. Let the artwork be a visual mirror of your spirit.

WHAT YOU NEED

⇒ Paper or canvas

⇒ Paint and brush

⇒ Markers

⇒ Collage materials

THERAPIST'S INSIGHT

Your differences and strengths can be your superpower. We know that people with ADHD who are aware of their strengths will have better mental health – this exercise boosts self-esteem and emotional resilience.

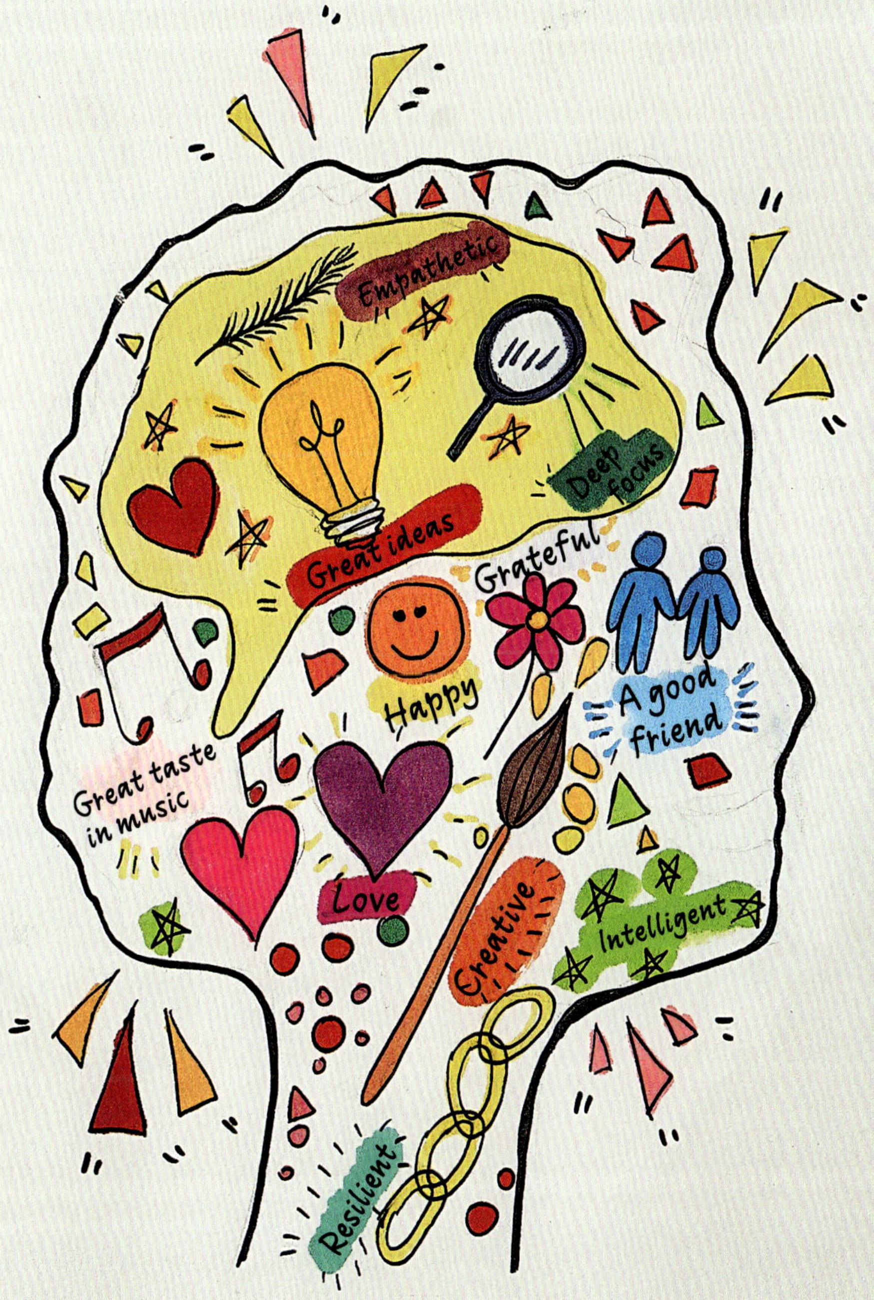
Empathetic
Deep focus
Great ideas
Grateful
Happy
A good friend
Great taste in music
Love
Creative
Intelligent
Resilient

EXERCISE 34

Sensory collage

Using colour, texture and layering can make your senses feel calm and support creative enquiry. It helps turn tactile exploration into a soothing, intentional process.

INSTRUCTIONS

1. Collect textured or colourful scraps you feel drawn to.
2. Cut or tear them into shapes that feel right.
3. Glue them onto your page, layering them as you go.
4. Let your fingers explore the textures.
5. Add drawn or painted details, if you like.

WHAT YOU NEED

⇛ Paper

⇛ Textured materials (fabric, tissue, ribbon, card)

⇛ Scissors

⇛ Glue

⇛ Pen or paint and brush (optional)

THERAPIST'S INSIGHT

Exploring the sense of touch can help people manage uncomfortable sensations, quiet the nervous system and increase focus. Be aware of how you feel during and after this exercise – and if you are overwhelmed, return to using touch to ground you.

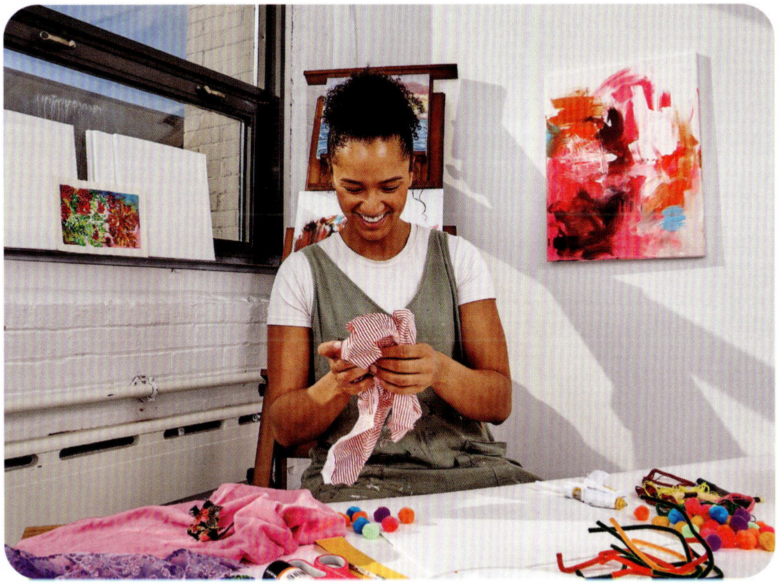

Step 1

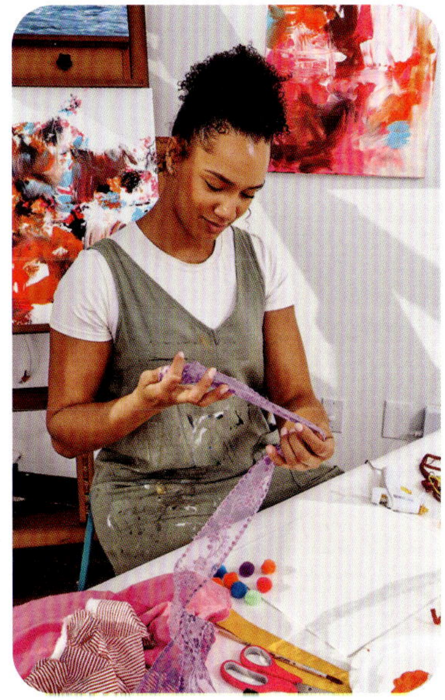

Step 4

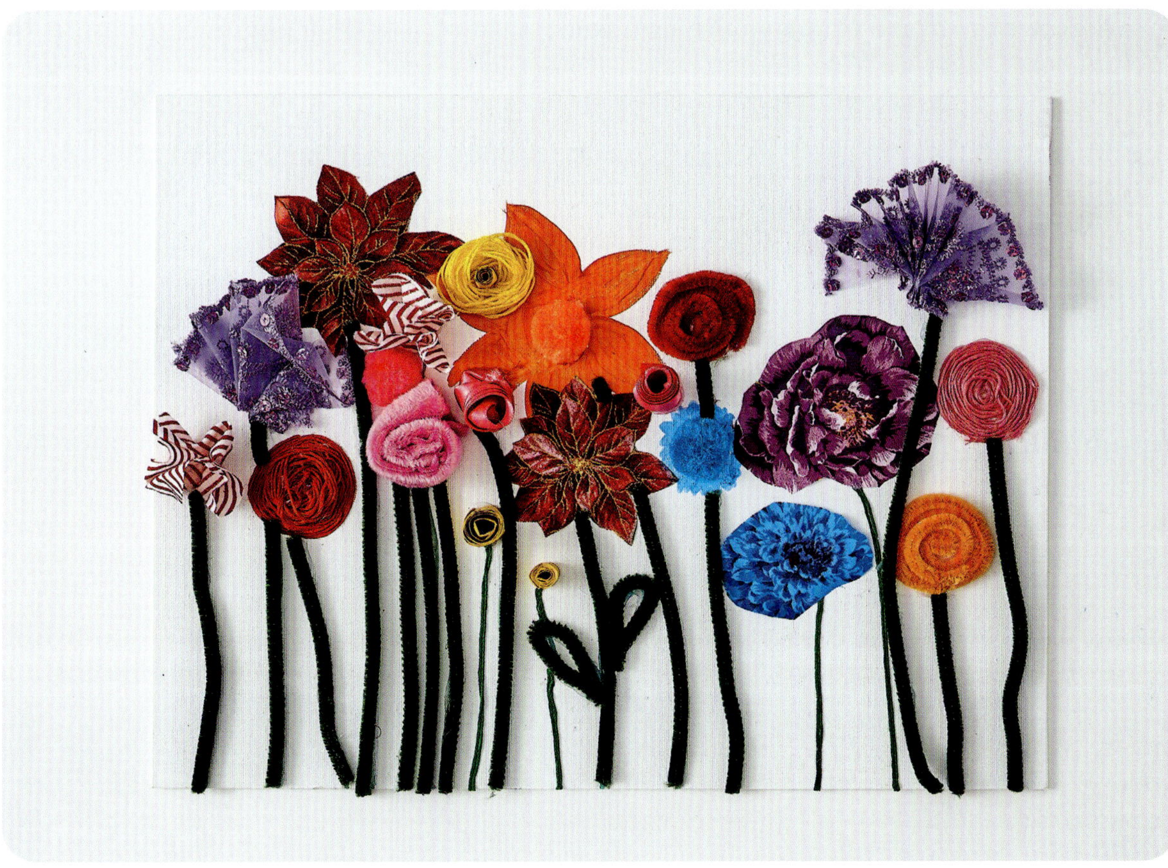

EXERCISE 35

Feeling to flow

Using sound, scent or texture to inspire a drawing strengthens cross-sensory creativity. It encourages play and celebrates unique ways of experiencing the world.

INSTRUCTIONS

1. Choose one sensory focus – a song, a scent or a textured object.
2. Decide how these things make you feel.
3. Begin drawing or painting that feeling, rather than capturing its literal form.
4. Let the energy guide your strokes.
5. Stop when the emotion feels fully expressed.

WHAT YOU NEED

- ⇛ Paper
- ⇛ Music or an object with texture/scent
- ⇛ Pencils or paint and brush

THERAPIST'S INSIGHT

'Numbing out' is a survival device whereby the nervous system feels numb or shuts down in response to sensory or emotional overload. By isolating a single sense, we can regulate this sensory overwhelm and move towards a more relaxed and regulated state.

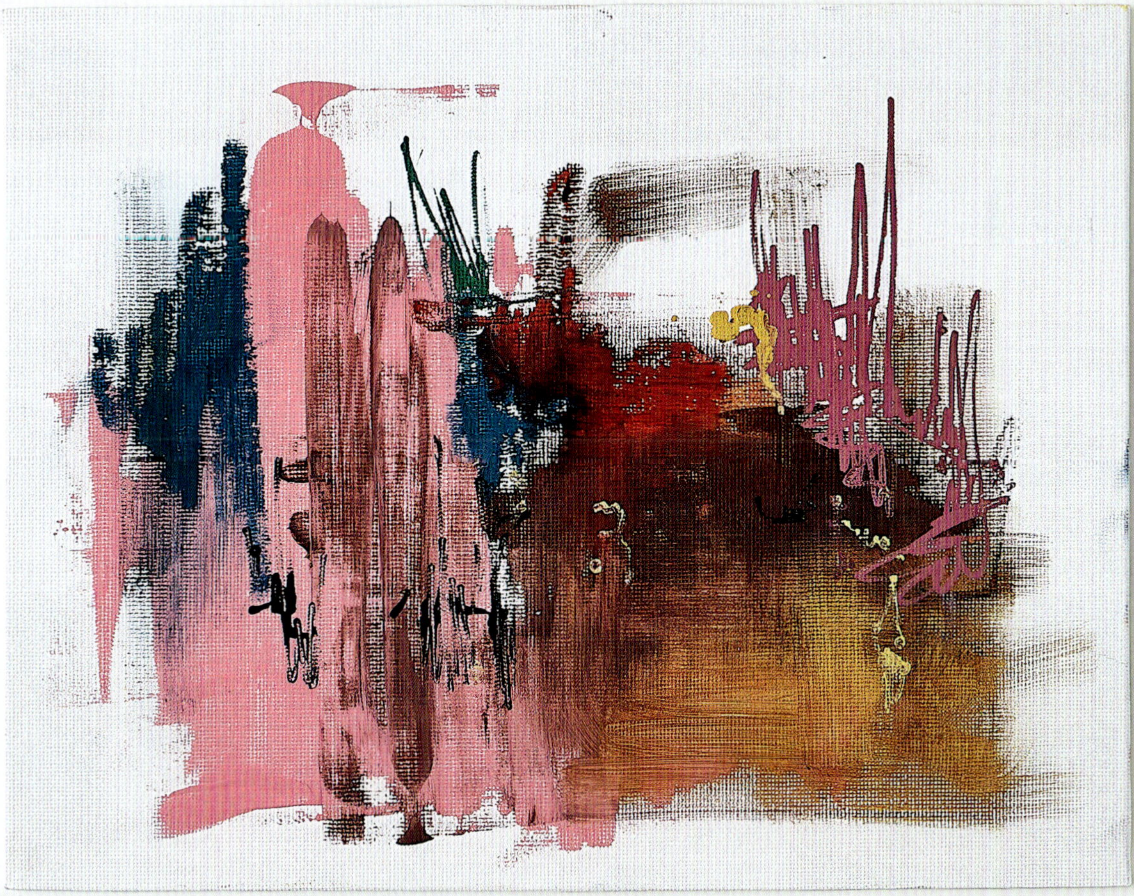

EXERCISE 36

Hyperfocus drawing

Hyperfocus can be helpful when used with care, as it becomes a form of flow. This exercise channels that deep attention into gentle mindfulness and an appreciation for detail.

INSTRUCTIONS

1. Choose one small object – a shell, button or leaf.
2. Look closely at its details, edges, shadows and texture.
3. Begin drawing slowly, capturing what you see.
4. Stay with the drawing until you feel a sense of stillness.
5. Let your focus feel spacious, not pressured.

WHAT YOU NEED

⇛ Paper

⇛ A small object of your choice

⇛ Fine pen or pencil

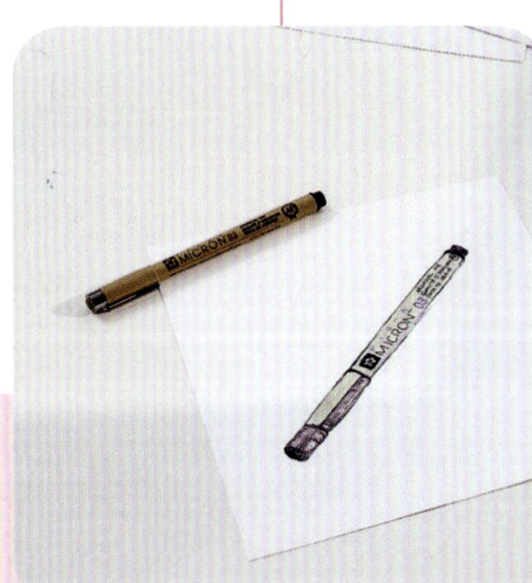

Alternative drawing

THERAPIST'S INSIGHT

Focusing on one single thing creates a low-stimulation environment, helping combat feelings of overwhelm. This hyperfocus can help you enter a state of deep, effortless absorption, increasing creativity and reducing anxiety.

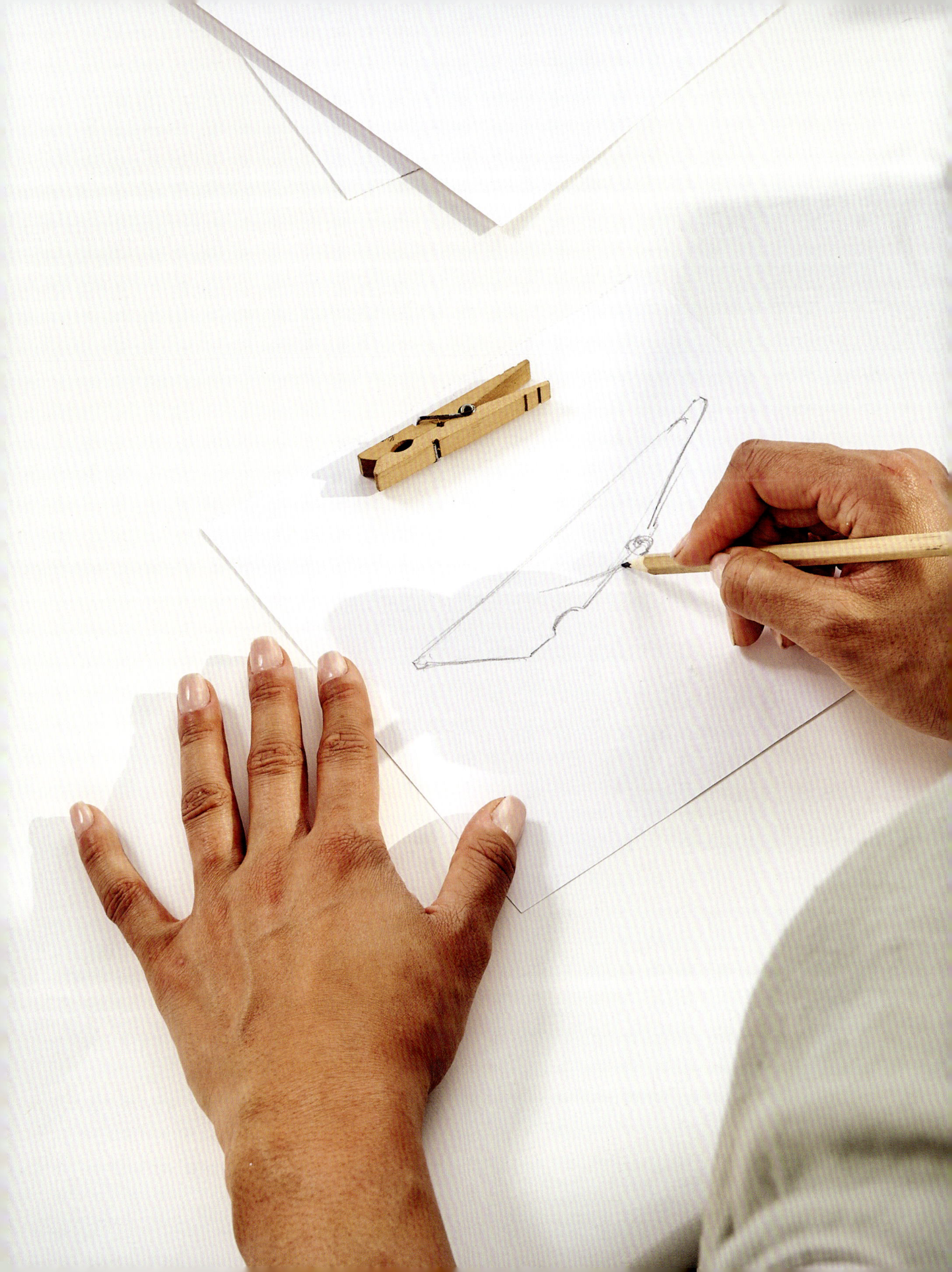

EXERCISE 37

Routine mandala

This exercise combines creativity with structure, using a traditional mandala as a visual way to organize your day. It is especially helpful if your mind feels busy or easily distracted. It gives your thoughts a place to land while still encouraging creativity and flexibility.

INSTRUCTIONS

1. Draw a mandala in the centre of your page. It doesn't need to be perfect or symmetrical – just draw in a way that feels natural.
2. Once your central shape is complete, add sections that branch out from the mandala.
3. In each section, write down things you'd like to do today that ground you. These can be small, simple things or bigger priorities.
4. Add colour, patterns, or marks to each section. Let this part feel calm and intuitive.

WHAT YOU NEED

⇛ Paper

⇛ Your favourite art materials – anything you enjoy using

⇛ Pencil or pen

THERAPIST'S INSIGHT

A structured routine can help focus attention for those with ADHD, while the consistency removes sensory unpredictability, helping reduce stress hormones. Turning your routine into a work of art creates a visual support, helping you to anticipate upcoming activities and support emotional regulation as a result.

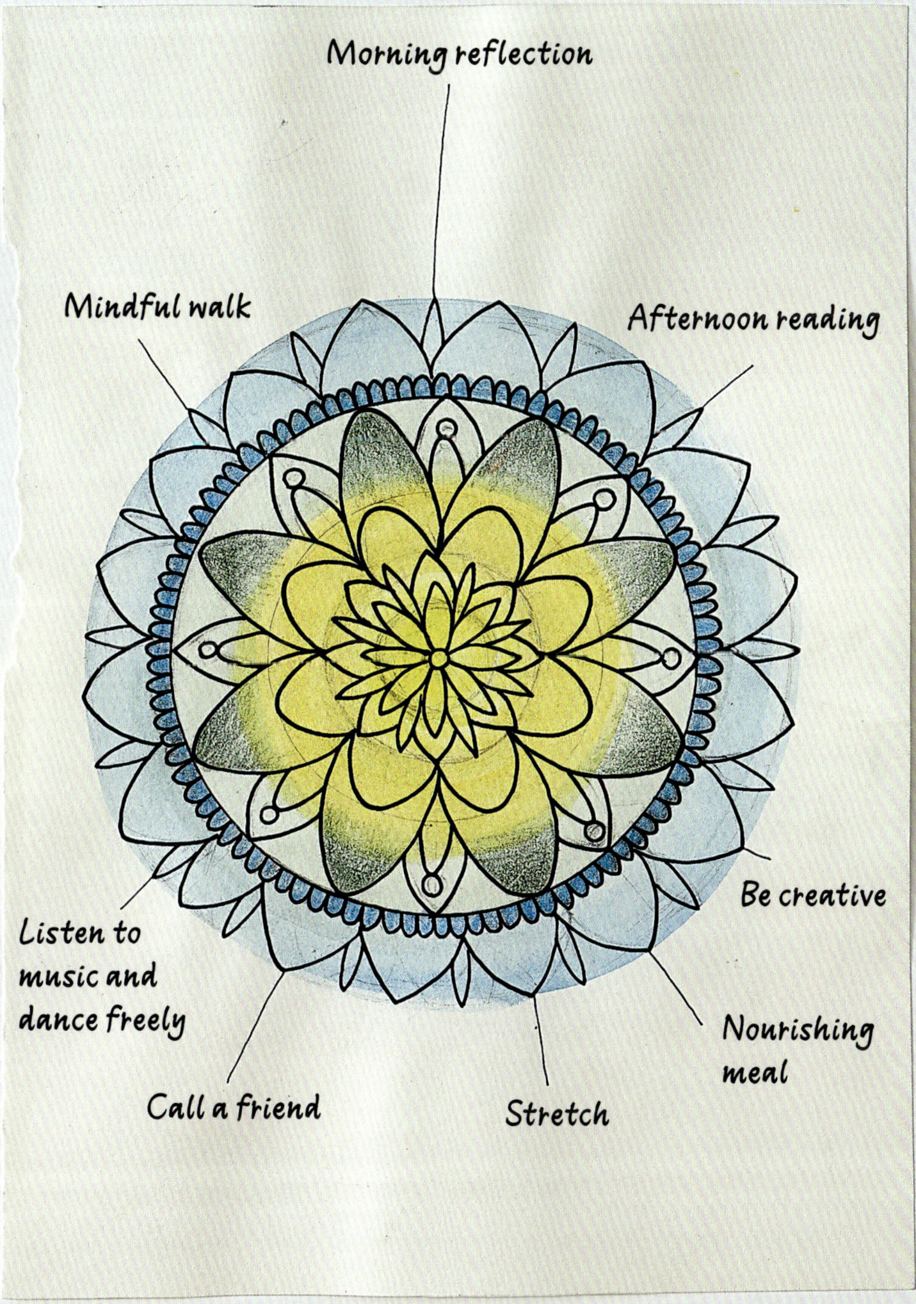
Morning reflection
Mindful walk
Afternoon reading
Be creative
Listen to music and dance freely
Nourishing meal
Call a friend
Stretch

EXERCISE 38

Hidden message layer

Many neurodivergent people struggle to express feelings out loud or in front of others – not because they do not feel deeply, but because they feel too deeply.

This exercise allows you to express the emotion privately, without feeling vulnerable.

INSTRUCTIONS

1. Write a sentence or word expressing how you feel.
2. Cover it with layers of abstract marks, shapes or paint until it disappears.
3. Now only you know what lies beneath.
4. Add shimmer or gold over the top as a symbol of release.

WHAT YOU NEED

- ⇛ Paper
- ⇛ Pen
- ⇛ Coloured pens or pencils, or paint and brush
- ⇛ Shimmer or gold pen or paint

THERAPIST'S INSIGHT

This exercise gives you permission to take a break from masking your emotions and be true to how you are feeling. It can help you relax and restore your energy. It is also a reminder that you don't need to change anything about yourself.

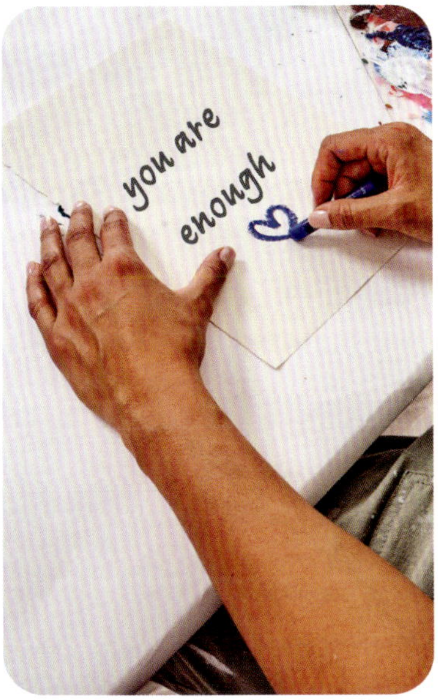

Step 1

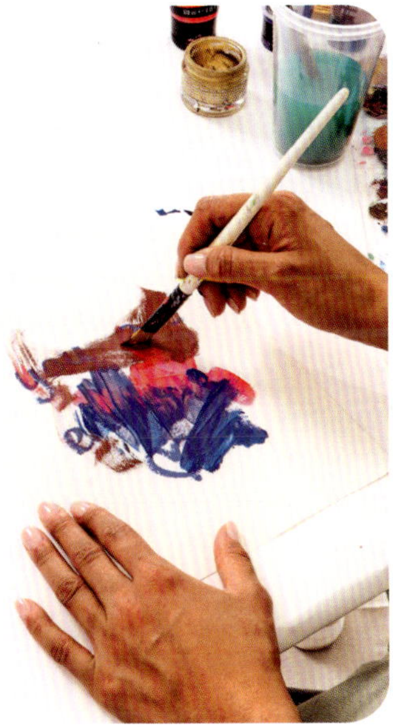
Step 2

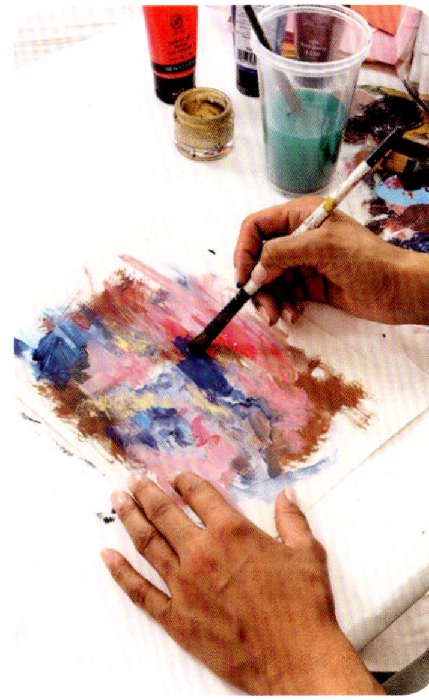
Step 4

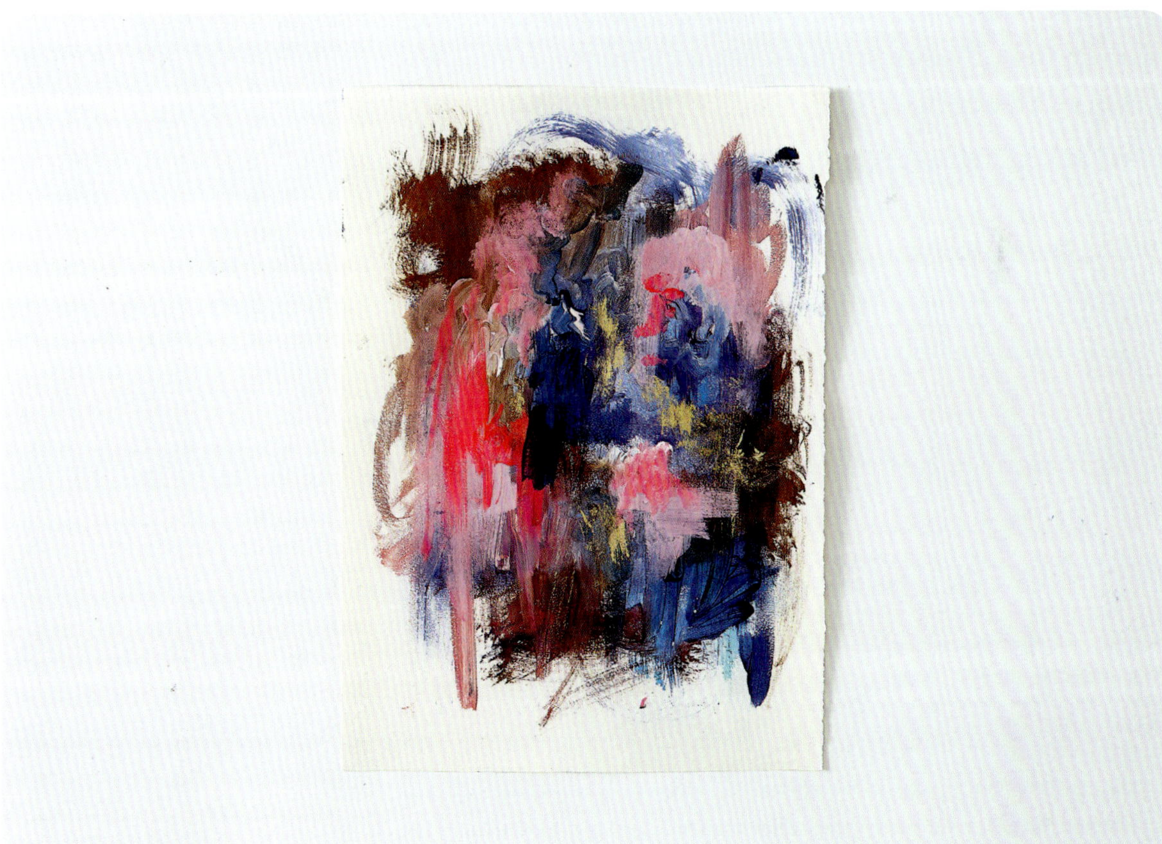

EXERCISE 39

Touch & trace

This exercise lets you zero in on your body rather than your thoughts by anchoring your focus in tactile sensation. This interrupts the pattern of overthinking, mental noise or creative paralysis common to neurodivergent people.

WHAT YOU NEED

- ⇒ Paper
- ⇒ A pen or soft pencil
- ⇒ A small textured object (a leaf, shell, pine cone or stone)

INSTRUCTIONS

1. Hold a textured object in one hand. Close your eyes if that feels safe. Slowly run your fingers over the object's surface – notice every bump, curve or edge.
2. With your other hand, begin to draw what the texture *feels* like. Let your hand move in rhythm with the sensation – rough becomes jagged lines, smooth becomes long sweeps, soft becomes circular or blurred marks.
3. When you're done, open your eyes and take a moment to notice how your body feels.

THERAPIST'S INSIGHT

Sensory processing can be challenging for neurodivergent people, as they may feel sensations too strongly or not strongly enough. Limiting sensory input and focusing deeply on touch helps reduce overstimulation and supports the brain's reward system.

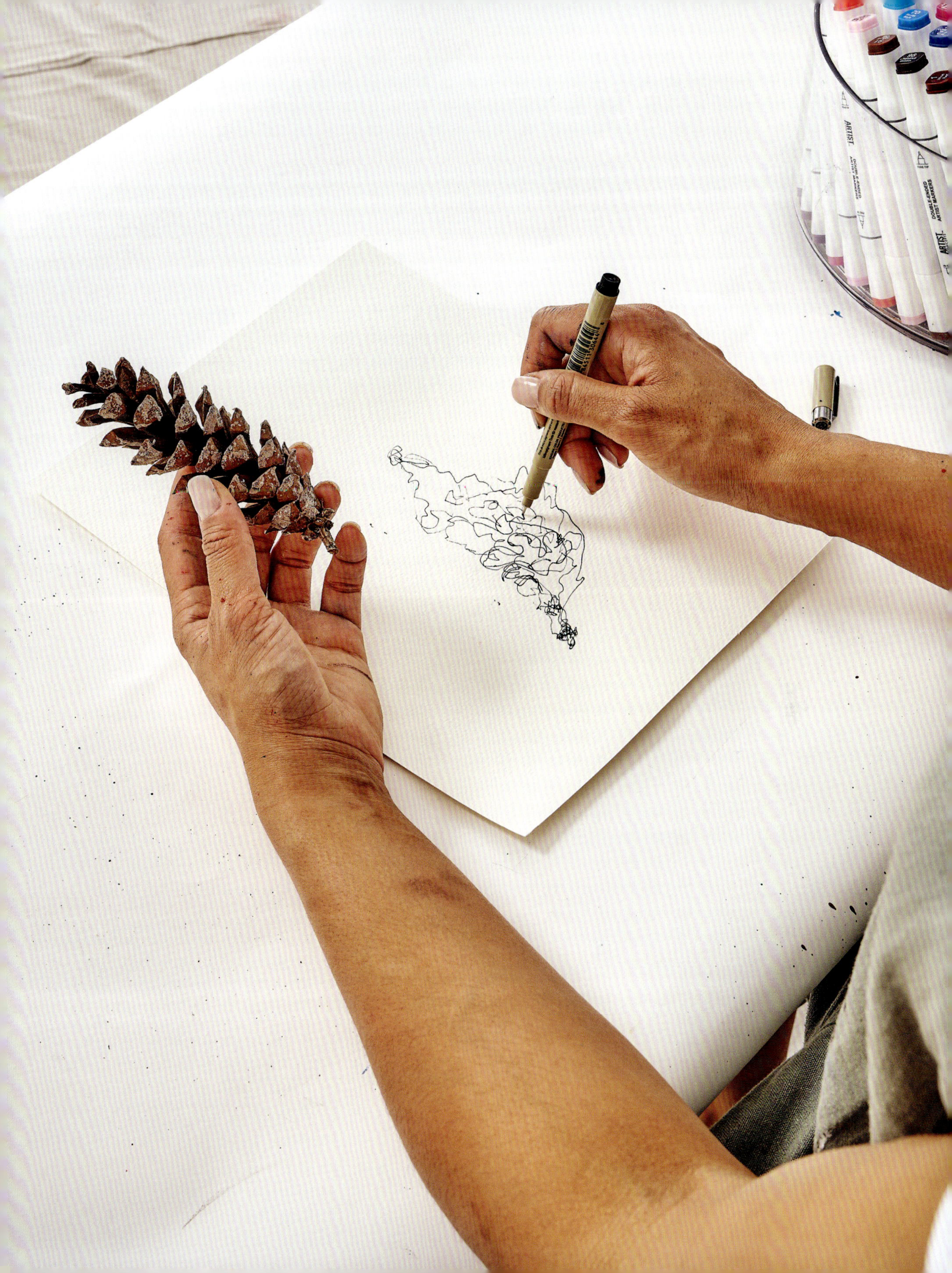

EXERCISE 40

Sound shapes

Translating what you hear into shapes develops sensory awareness and creative flexibility. It stimulates multiple senses and encourages spontaneous expression.

INSTRUCTIONS

1. Listen carefully to sounds around you, or play a song.
2. Use your choice of materials to draw shapes that match each sound's energy or pitch.
3. Let high sounds be shown by light lines, and low sounds by heavy or bold ones.
4. Fill the page intuitively.
5. Observe how sound has taken form on paper.

WHAT YOU NEED

- ⇒ Paper
- ⇒ Music or environmental sounds
- ⇒ Your favourite art materials – anything you enjoy using

THERAPIST'S INSIGHT

Creating an environment where sensory experiences are seen within a larger, harmonious whole helps the brain absorb them more effectively. In this way they can become useful rather than overwhelming.

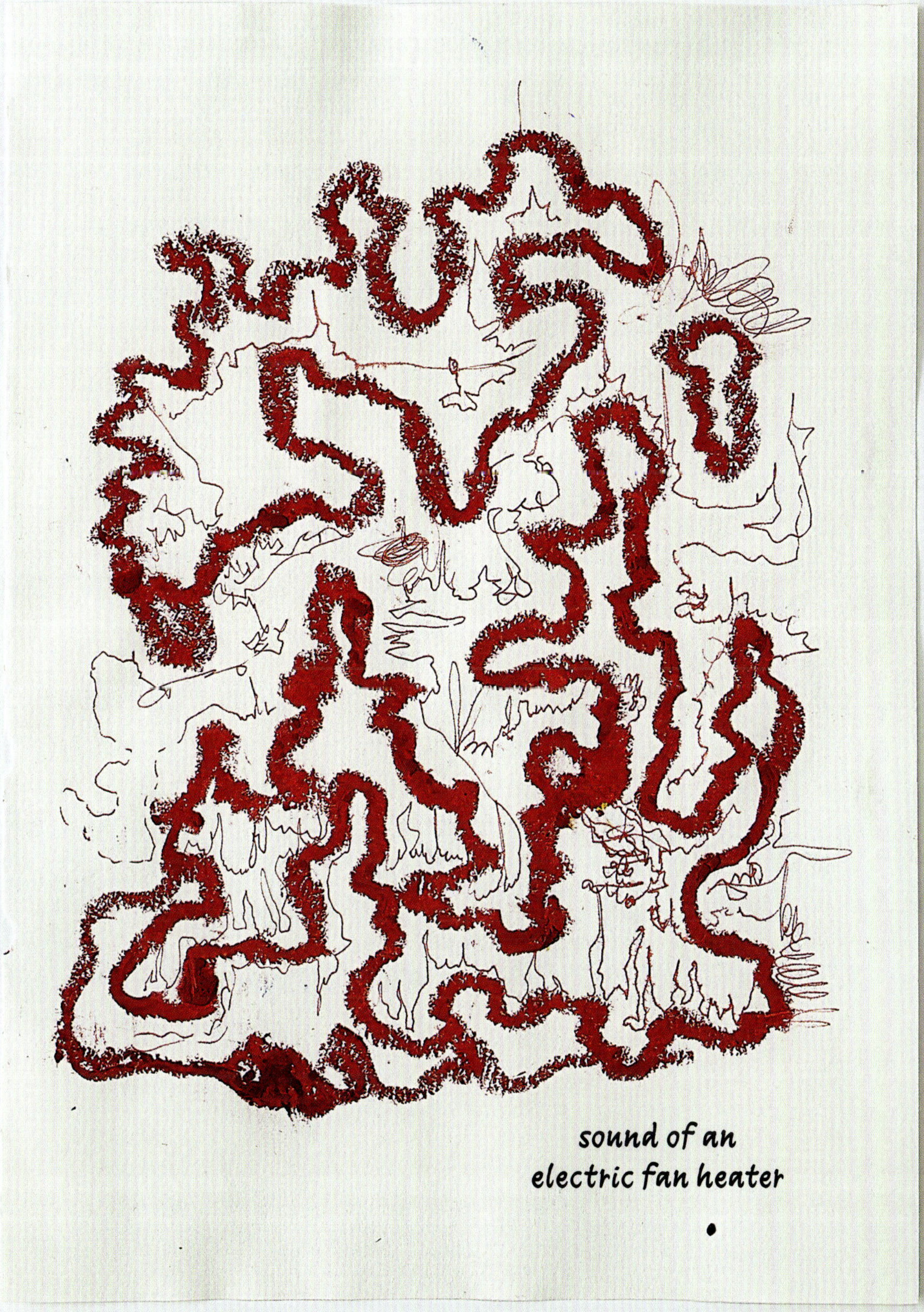

sound of an
electric fan heater

EXERCISE 41

Three-tool challenge

Neurodivergent brains often struggle with *too many choices* – which tool, which colour, which technique and what to do next. This exercise shows how a restricted choice can bring freedom. Limiting the options to just three tools can create instant calm, and this helps reduce mental noise.

INSTRUCTIONS

1. Create an abstract art piece using the three tools you have chosen.

WHAT YOU NEED

- Paper or canvas
- Three tools of your choice, such as a palette knife, a brush and an everyday item
- Art materials you enjoy using with these tools, such as ink or acrylic paint

THERAPIST'S INSIGHT

This exercise gives limited choices, which allows the neurodivergent brain to experience a sense of calm. This encourages a flow state by directing energy along one clear path, helping reduce stress and anxiety.

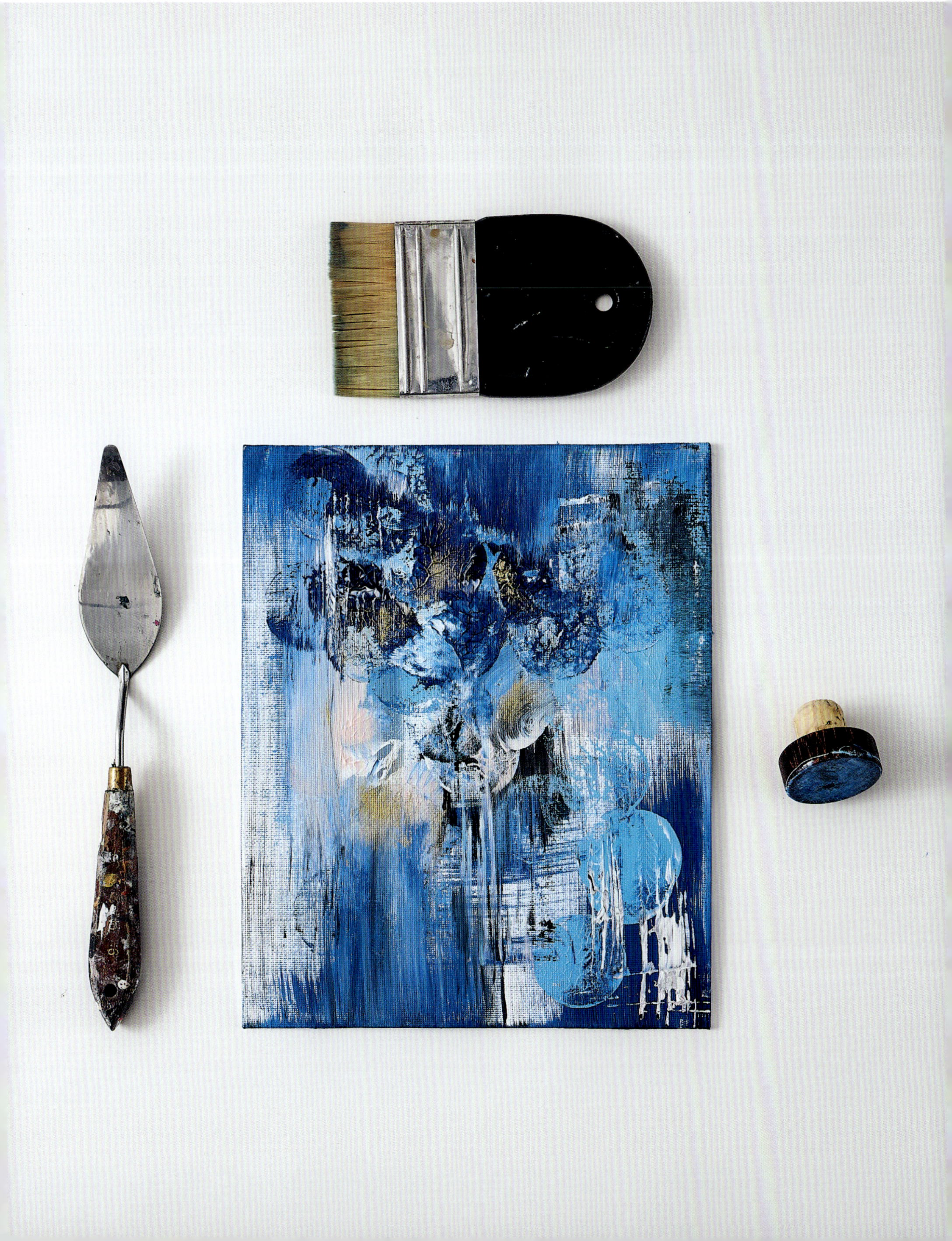

EXERCISE 42

Pixel pieces

Breaking big tasks into smaller 'pixels' or squares mirrors how neurodivergent minds process detail. It encourages patience and focus, and gives satisfaction from taking small steps.

WHAT YOU NEED

- ⇒ Graph paper or gridded page
- ⇒ Object of your choice
- ⇒ Pens or markers

INSTRUCTIONS

1. Choose an individual object, such as the orange used here. Choose colours to fit and make shapes to fill the grid on your paper.
2. Colour one small square (pixel) at a time.
3. Work slowly, section by section.
4. Notice how each tiny square helps build the bigger picture.
5. Stop whenever the rhythm of the shapes feels soothing.

THERAPIST'S INSIGHT

Having clear, small goals allows the brain to experience multiple rewards. Working in this way, pixel by pixel, means that you will eventually have the gratification of completing a larger task. This triggers dopamine release, reinforcing positive behaviour and increasing motivation.

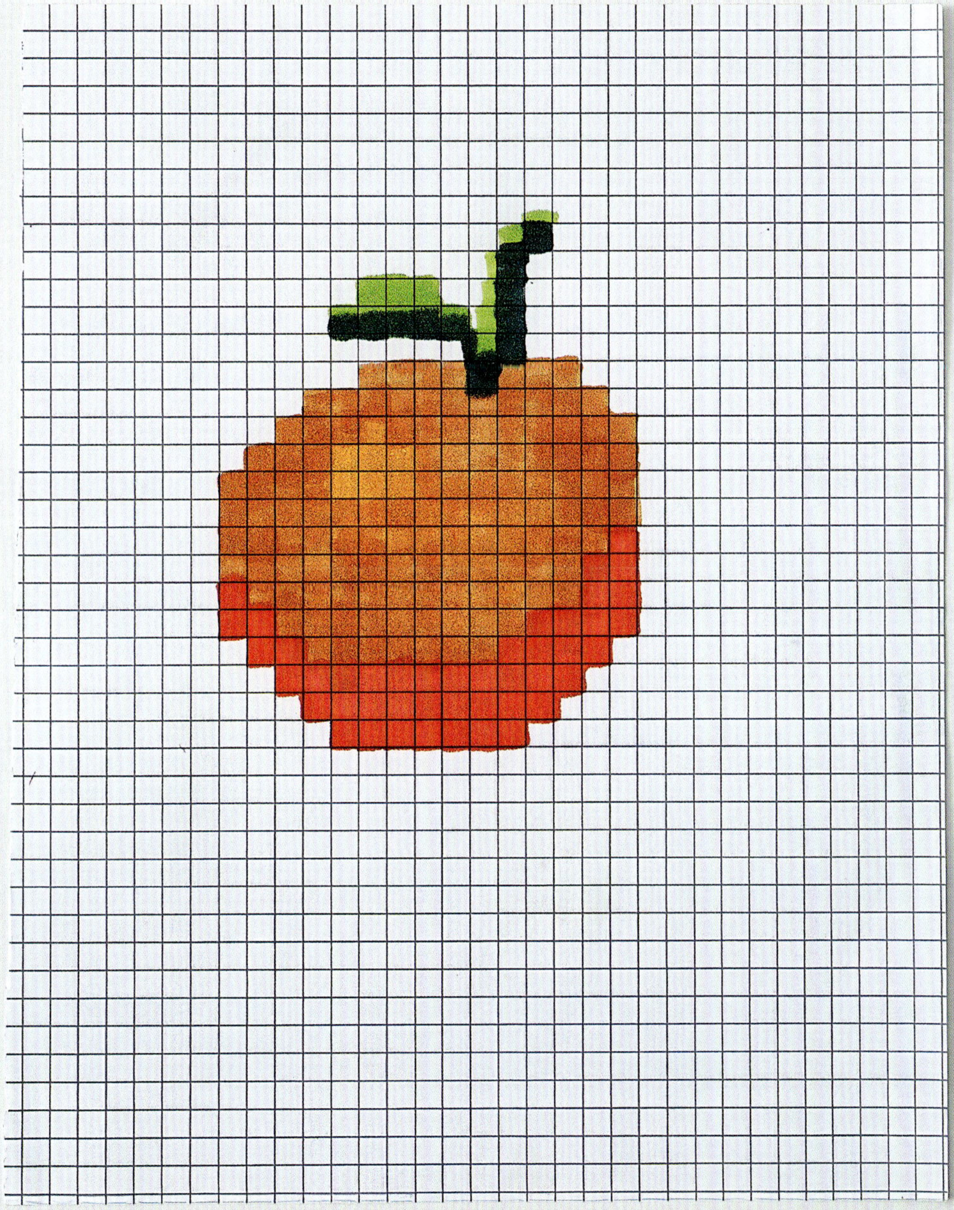

EXERCISE 43

Stained-glass emotions

This exercise turns complex emotions into smaller, manageable parts, representing them through colour and shape on the page. This helps to reduce overwhelm.

INSTRUCTIONS

1. Draw random curving and intersecting lines across the page with a pencil or pen.
2. Consider how you are feeling right now and assign a colour to each feeling. For example, yellow could represent joy while blue might represent calm.
3. Colour each segment created by the intersecting lines based on how you feel – there are no rules.
4. Use a dark marker to trace over the lines to make each section stand out more.

WHAT YOU NEED

- ⇛ Paper
- ⇛ Coloured pens or pencils, including a dark marker

THERAPIST'S INSIGHT

Attunement is a term in psychology that refers to becoming aware of, and connected with, your own limits, and recognizing your emotions. This exercise encourages this awareness, allowing you to understand what you need to stay calm and grounded.

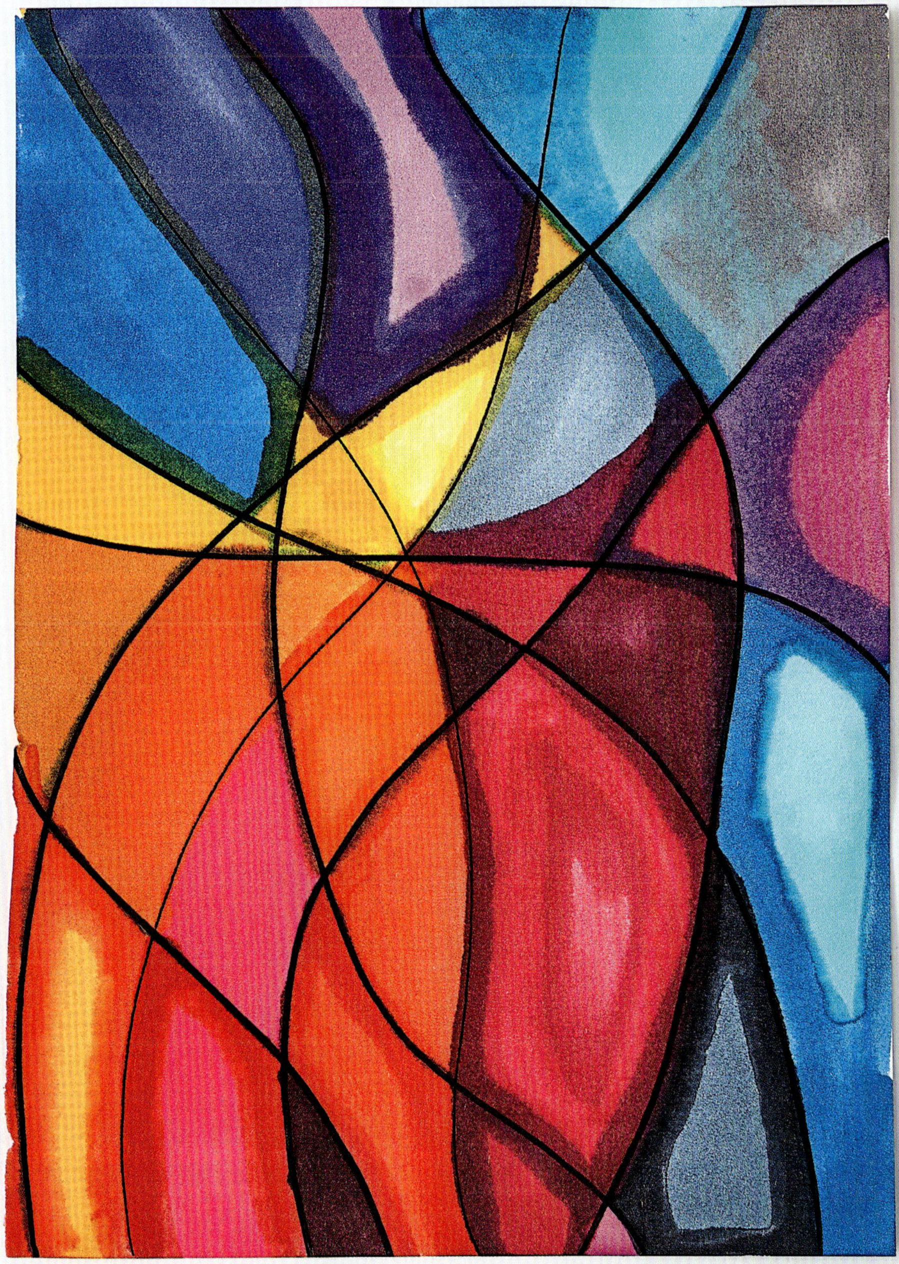

CHAPTER 5

HOPE, JOY & REFLECTION

Introduction

After practising grounding, letting go and sitting with uncertainty, there is often space for something lighter to emerge – moments of hope, quiet joy or gentle reflection. This chapter is a reminder that creativity can hold space not only for processing and release, but also for renewal, meaning and gentle optimism. These feelings may show up subtly, as ease, softness or a renewed sense of connection.

The exercises in this chapter encourage you to explore colour, rhythm and mark-making in ways that feel expansive rather than contained. Reflection is an important part of this process. Take time to acknowledge your experience and notice how your relationship with creativity – and with yourself – may have changed.

For neurodivergent minds, joy can sometimes feel fleeting or undeserved, especially after long periods of stress or overwhelm. This chapter reminds you that joy does not need to be earned. It can exist alongside difficulty. It can be simple, quiet and momentary – and still be real.

As you move through these pages, allow yourself to notice what feels hopeful, nourishing and alive. These reflections can become anchors – small reminders that you can return to when you need reassurance or light.

THERAPIST'S NOTE

Hope and joy are emotions to recognize as they are experienced. 'Resourcing' is a practice in Emotion Focused Therapy (EFT) where you build a sense of safety, calm and strength within yourself by reflecting on gratitude, grounding yourself in the present or reframing your experiences in a positive way. Connecting with positive experiences and fostering hope and joy is a powerful skill to work on because it helps change how your brain and nervous system respond. The brain is shaped by its regular habits, so as you practise gratitude and positivity, these emotions will become more accessible. Reflecting on positive moments activates the part of the brain connected to memory and reward, helping to decrease stress and calm your nervous system. Reminding yourself that positive and joyful moments exist alongside other emotions helps to build resilience, self-compassion and connections to other people.

EXERCISE 44

Gratitude spiral

Acknowledging what you are thankful for rewires the brain to focus on safety and positivity. Creating this in the form of a spiral gives a visual reminder that gratitude expands endlessly and that saying 'thank you' helps to bring calm focus.

INSTRUCTIONS

1. In a notepad, write down a few things you are grateful for. Set the notepad aside.
2. On a piece of paper, draw a loose spiral starting from the centre of the page.
3. Decorate the spiral using colour, symbols, shapes and patterns that are special to you and relate to the things you are grateful for.
4. When finished, sit with your gratitude spiral. Display it somewhere prominent to remind you daily of the things you are grateful for.

WHAT YOU NEED

⇛ Notepad

⇛ Paper

⇛ Art materials you enjoy using

THERAPIST'S INSIGHT

By representing gratitude in a visual form, you might find it easier to stay connected to this emotion. Gratitude is a powerful tool for rewiring the brain and creating new positive neural pathways. The more you practise gratitude, the more you'll start to notice and feel it.

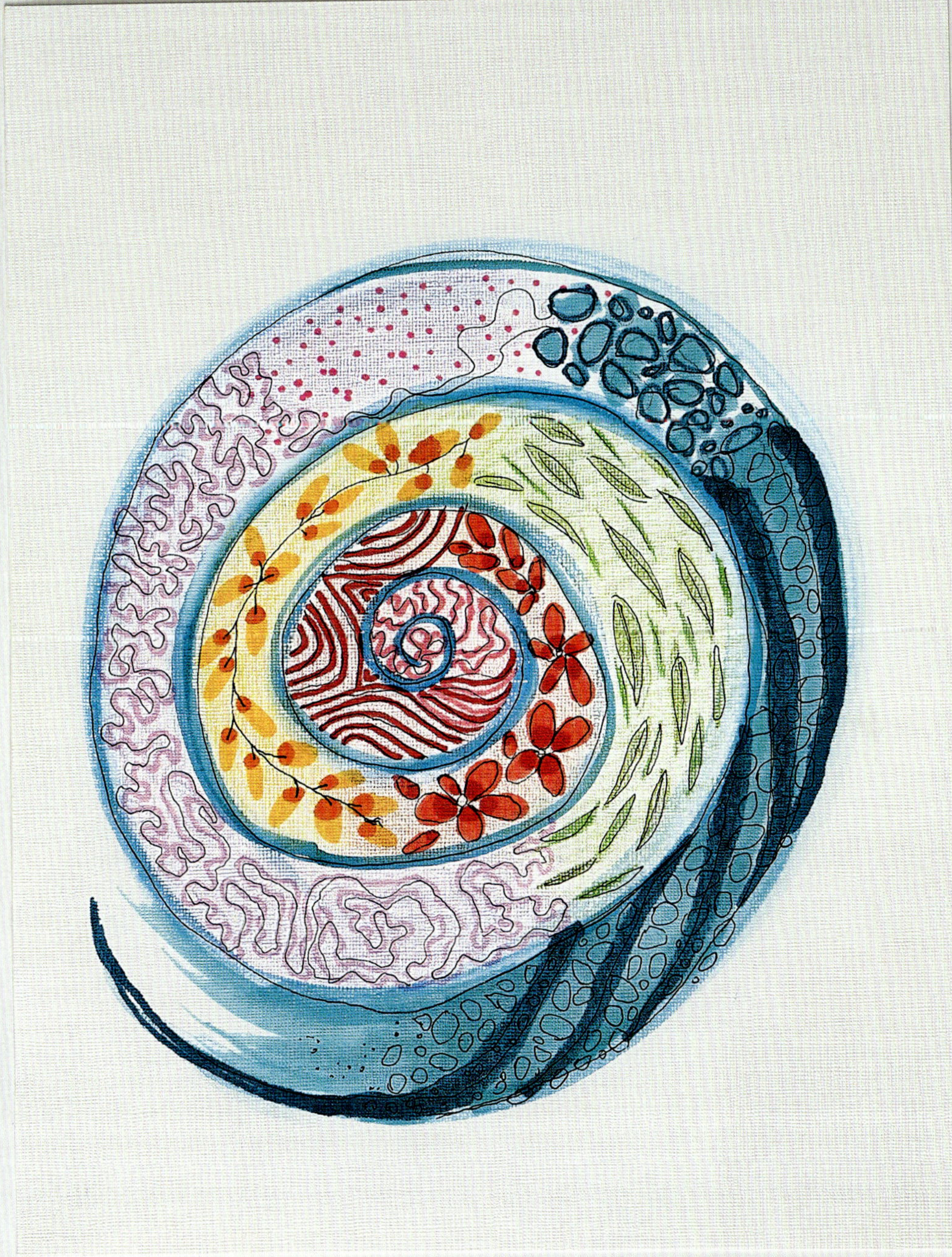

EXERCISE 45

Future window

Visualizing a positive future – whether symbolic or literal – helps the brain create hope. It strengthens belief in what is possible and helps shift focus from fear to faith.

INSTRUCTIONS

1. Draw the outline of a window frame – it can be any shape you like.
2. Inside the frame, draw or paint what you hope to see in your future.
3. Think about how that vision feels, not just how it looks.
4. Add colours that express warmth, joy or possibility.
5. Keep what you have created as a reminder of what you are growing towards.

WHAT YOU NEED

⇒ Paper

⇒ Pencil, or paint and brush

THERAPIST'S INSIGHT

This exercise is similar to a vision board and has clear psychological benefits. Making your aspirations and hopes achievable helps to strengthen positive expectations. This 'future window' can be a visual reminder of the hope and joy that are in store.

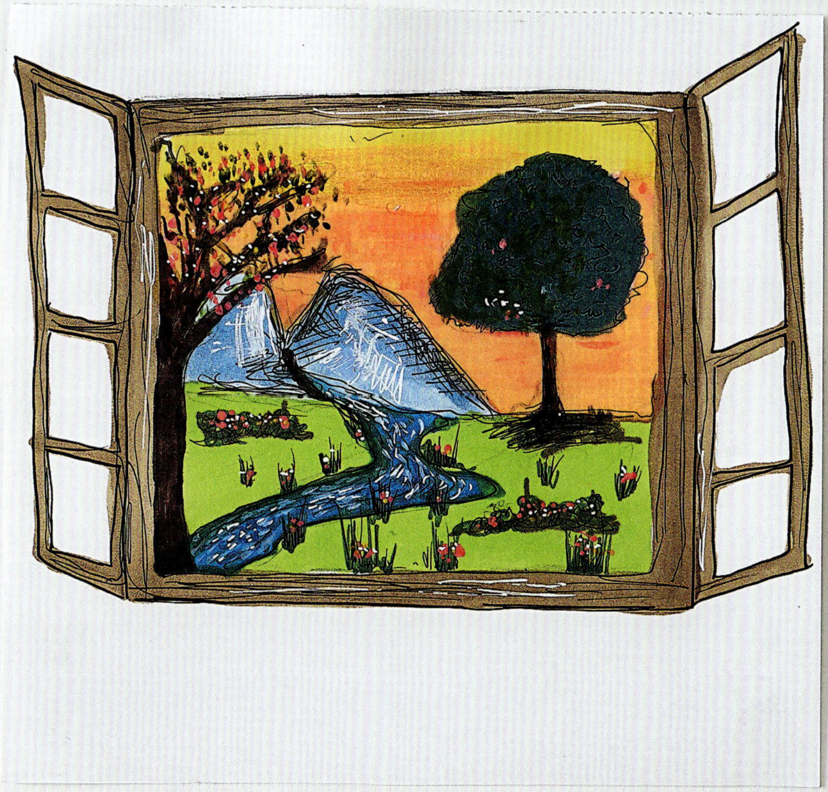

EXERCISE 46

Joyful colour bursts

Bright colours can lift your mood and create a sense of joy. Expressive splashes remind us that happiness can be spontaneous and playful.

INSTRUCTIONS

1. Choose vibrant paint or ink colours that make you feel joy.
2. Dilute the paint or ink with water so it is easier to flick.
3. Flick, tap or brush the colours freely onto your paper.
4. Let them overlap and mix.
5. Step back and notice the energy on the page.

WHAT YOU NEED

⇒ Paper

⇒ Bright paints or inks

⇒ Brushes or fingers

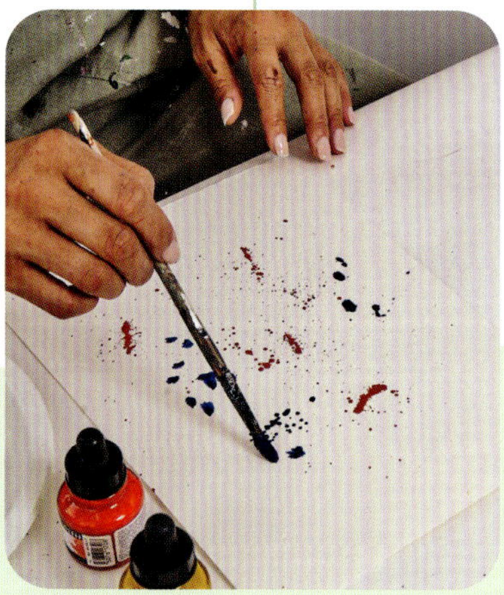

Step 3

THERAPIST'S INSIGHT

Colours can influence our emotions and attention, and vivid, joyful colours can help draw our focus to positive or hopeful moments. They can also make memories and emotional experiences more vivid and easier to recall.

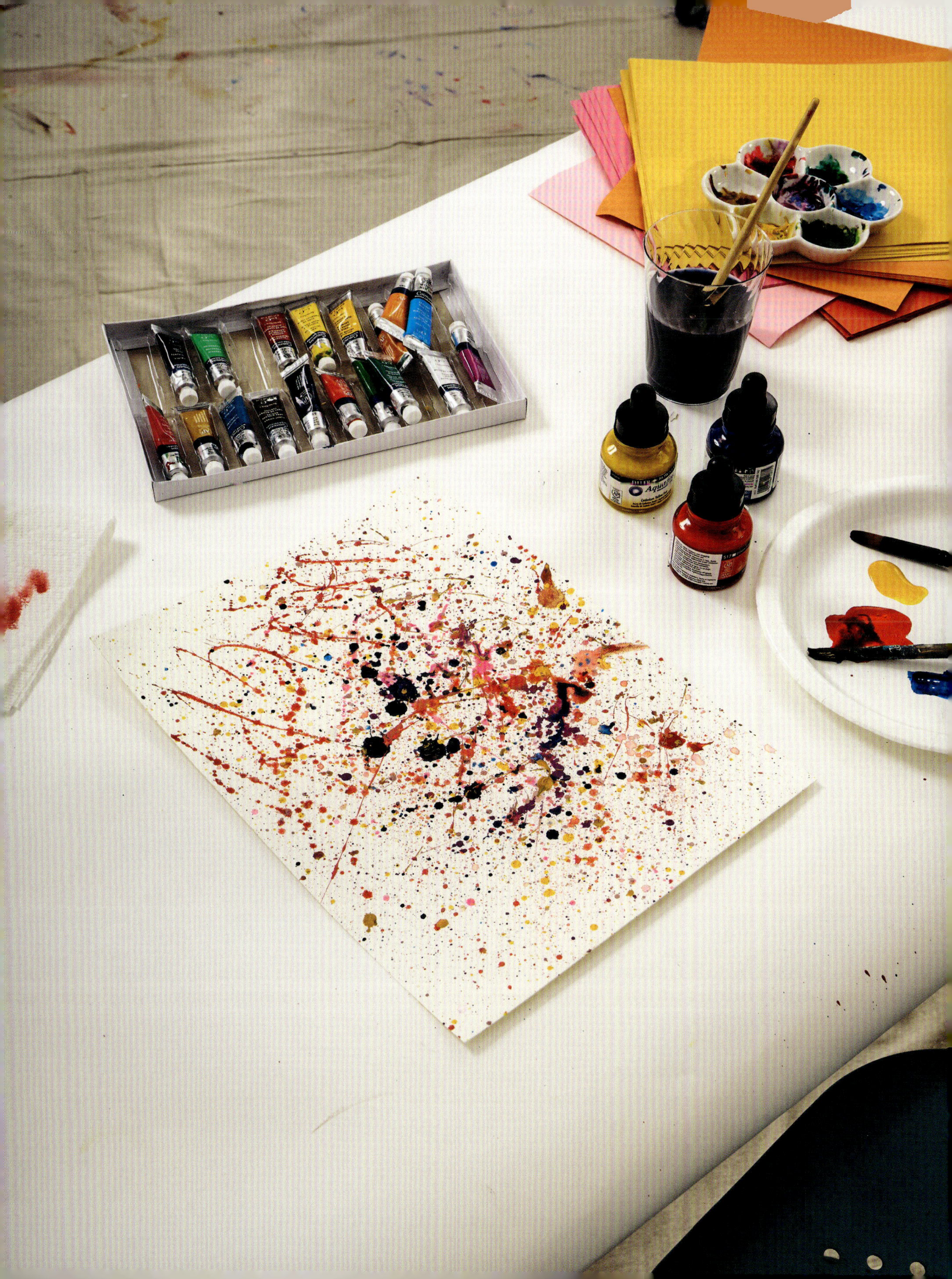

EXERCISE 47

Light rays

Drawing light reminds us of faith, renewal and inner strength. It connects you to something larger – creating a sense of divine warmth and hope.

INSTRUCTIONS

1. Start with a central point – your 'light source'.
2. Draw or paint rays around the central point, radiating outwards.
3. Layer soft colours to create a glowing effect.
4. Add symbols, words or soft textures, if you like.
5. Sit quietly in front of your finished piece for a moment of stillness.

WHAT YOU NEED

- ⇛ Paper
- ⇛ Yellow, gold or white paint, pencil or pastel
- ⇛ Brush (optional)

THERAPIST'S INSIGHT

The lightstream techinque focuses on a stream of light flowing towards and through the body, bringing healing and joyful energy. This exercise captures the essence of this technique, so focus on the feelings in your body as you create your own light rays on paper.

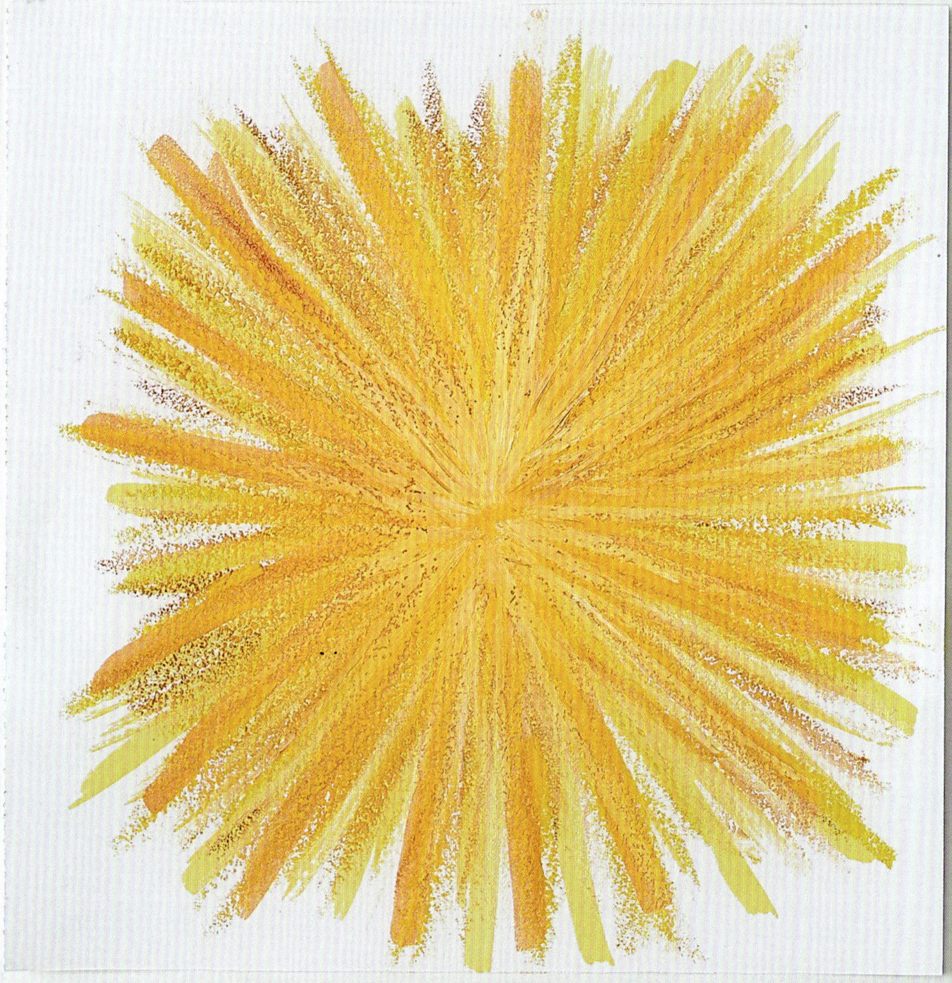

EXERCISE 48

Self-love doodles

Self-compassion strengthens resilience and softens the inner critic. For many neurodivergent people, kind thoughts can feel easier to sense than to say aloud.

When we turn self-love into visual marks, the nervous system can receive care without feeling any pressure or need to perform. The page becomes a gentle container for warmth, safety and reassurance.

INSTRUCTIONS

1. Before beginning, think of some loving or supportive messages that you could offer yourself. If helpful, write them down privately on a separate piece of paper. This is simply to set the emotional tone. Those feelings are then translated into colour, shape, movement and texture, rather than written words on the page. Let the messages guide your choice of colours, tools and movement.

WHAT YOU NEED

- Paper

A choice of media:

- Pen
- Paint and brush
- Coloured pencils
- Oil pastels
- Markers
- Watercolours

THERAPIST'S INSIGHT

This activity helps you see and understand yourself, creating feelings of safety. Developing this acceptance and openness to all parts of who you are builds resilience, helping you cope with criticism or hard moments.

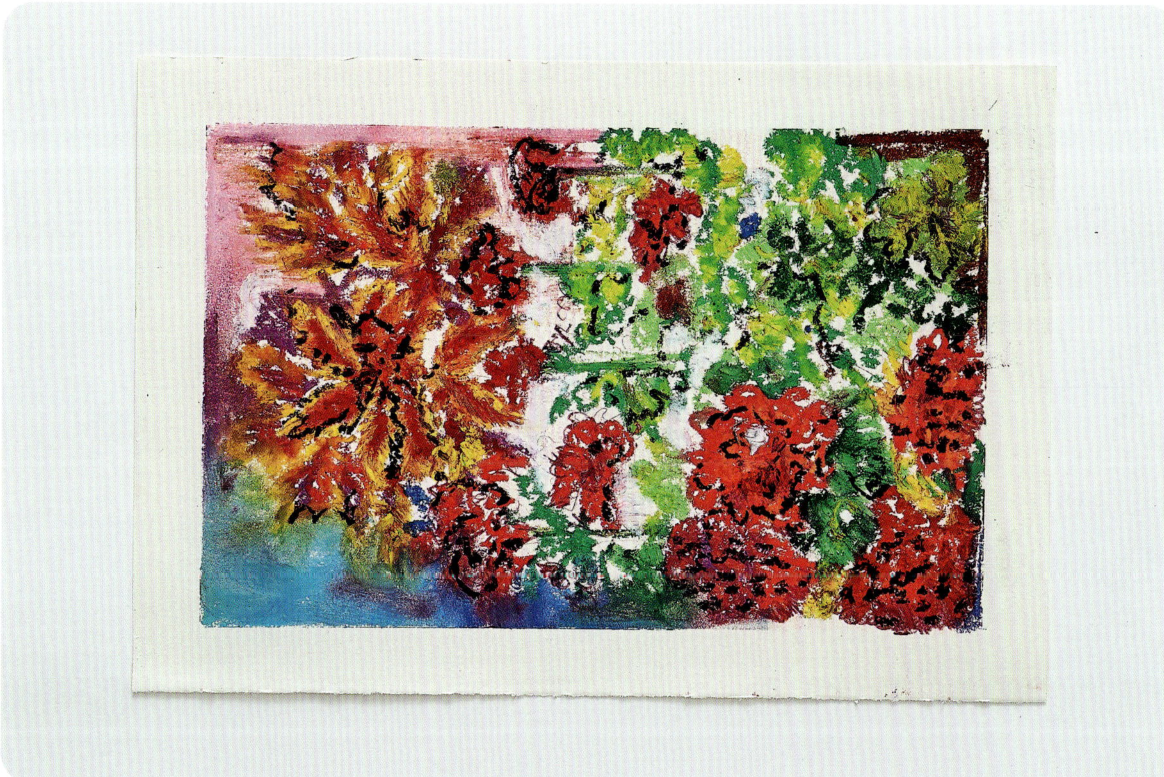

2. Begin with gentle marks, placing small doodles, shapes or flowing lines across the page. There is no focal point – let the kindness spread freely.

3. Use hearts, curves, flowers, spirals, dots or soft abstract shapes to represent care and encouragement.

4. Select colours that feel comforting or uplifting – tones that feel warm and supportive to you.

5. Fill the page gradually, allowing the page to become layered with softness. Stop when it feels complete.

AFFIRMATION
I meet myself
with tenderness.

EXERCISE 49

Mindset collage

Reflecting on positive memories, affirmations and words builds emotional resilience and strengthens your connection to joy, safety and love.

INSTRUCTIONS

1. Gather uplifting and encouraging images, affirmations or words from your materials.
2. Cut them out and arrange them on your page intuitively.
3. Glue them down and add doodles or notes around them, if you like.
4. Let the page represent empowerment.
5. Revisit what you have made whenever you need reassurance and encouragement.

WHAT YOU NEED

- ⇒ Paper
- ⇒ Old photos
- ⇒ Newspapers and magazines
- ⇒ Scissors
- ⇒ Glue
- ⇒ Pens or paint and brush (optional)

THERAPIST'S INSIGHT

Neurodivergent brains work harder to organize and plan, so creating art with existing images reduces the cognitive load. The repetition of cutting, gluing and sticking is similar to stimming and can help reduce stress levels.

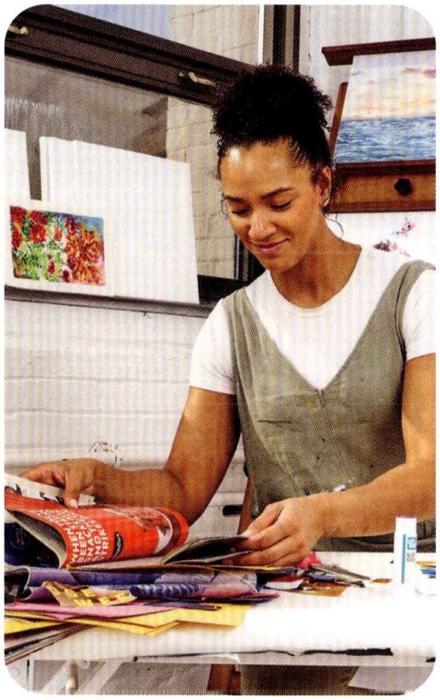
Step 1

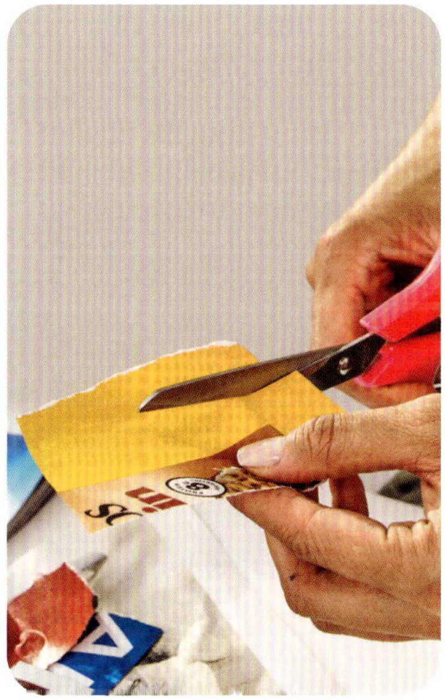
Step 2

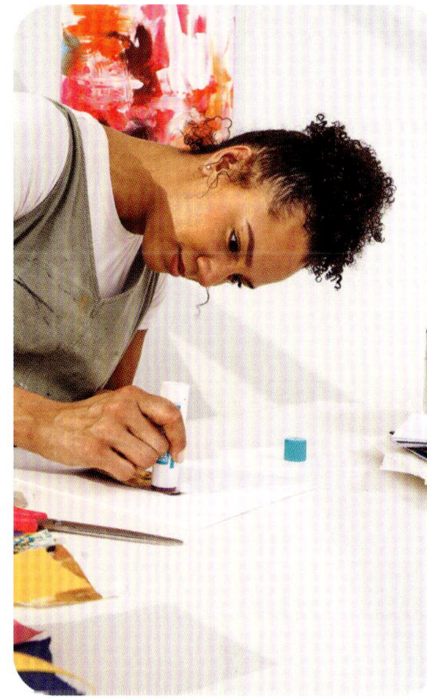
Step 3

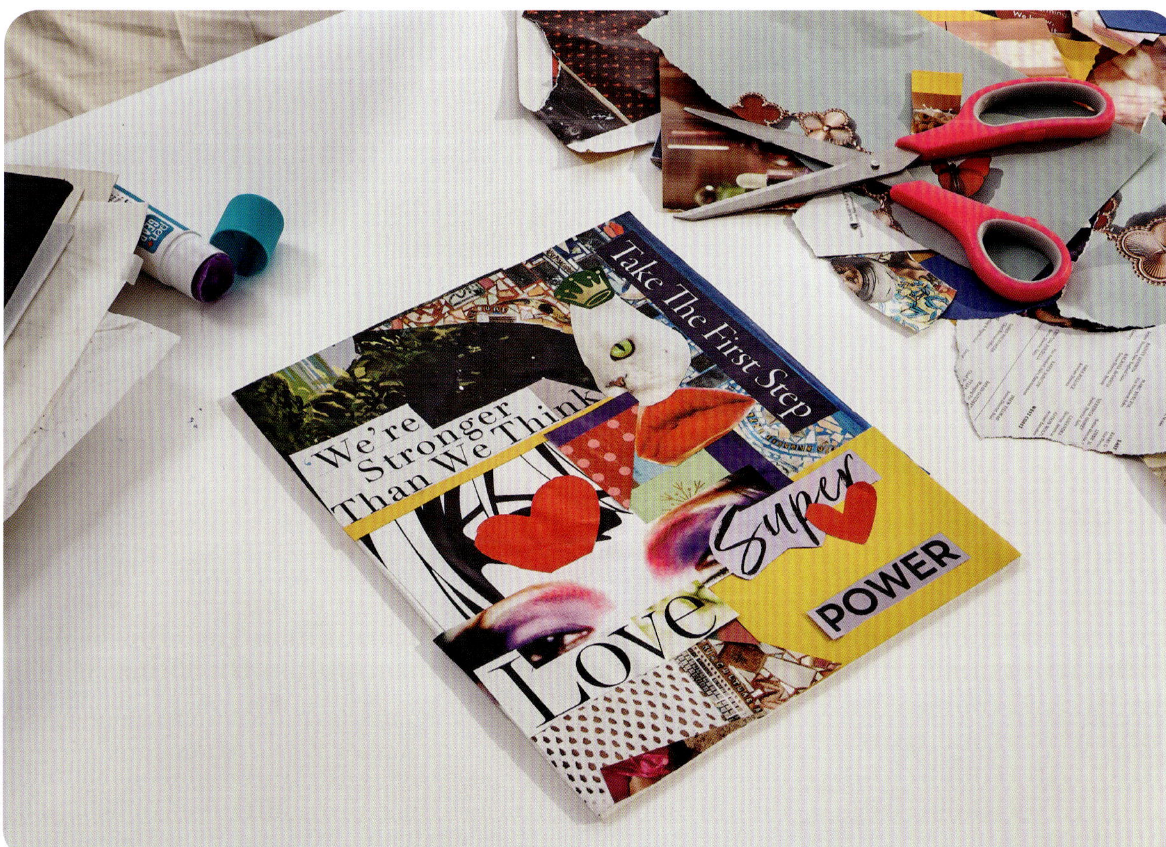

EXERCISE 50

Calm landscape

Visualizing peaceful environments can calm the nervous system and evoke feelings of safety. This exercise uses the imagination as a self-soothing tool.

INSTRUCTIONS

1. Think of a peaceful place – real or imaginary.
2. Begin drawing or painting it softly, focusing on calm colours and simple shapes.
3. Let the scene unfold naturally.
4. Add details like clouds, birds, the sun, trees or gentle waves, if you like.
5. Sit with the image quietly when it is done.

WHAT YOU NEED

⇛ Paper

⇛ Paint and brush or pencils

THERAPIST'S INSIGHT

The vagus nerve helps switch your body from stress into calm 'rest and digest' mode. This exercise signals to the vagus nerve that you are not in danger, helping your body shift into a state of relaxation and safety.

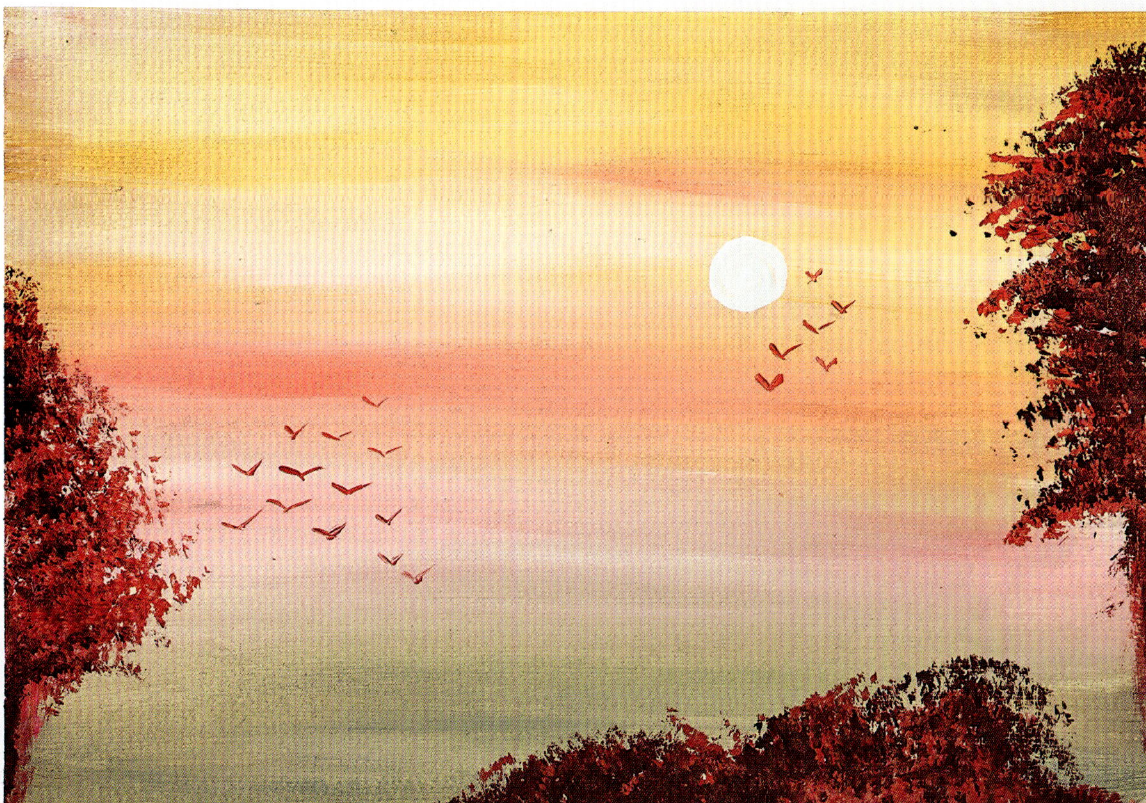

EXERCISE 51

Growth rings

Tree rings represent growth through time and the seasons. Creating them helps you see how your challenges have become layers of strength.

INSTRUCTIONS

1. In a notepad, write down the key personal growth points you are proud of. Set the notepad aside.
2. On a piece of paper, draw a spiral that starts in the centre of the page and expands outwards to reflect the growth rings of a tree. Each ring or colour represents a season, year or experience.
3. Add words or symbols that mark key growth points, if you wish. You can make this as colourful or simplistic as you wish.
4. Observe your 'tree of experience' with a sense of gratitude.

WHAT YOU NEED

- ⇛ Notepad
- ⇛ Paper
- ⇛ Pencil or paint and brush

THERAPIST'S INSIGHT

The rhythmic motion of drawing the same shape over and over is similar to stimming and helps the brain enter a relaxed flow state. Staying present as you draw can help reduce loud thoughts, creating a calm, meditative state and soothing the nervous system.

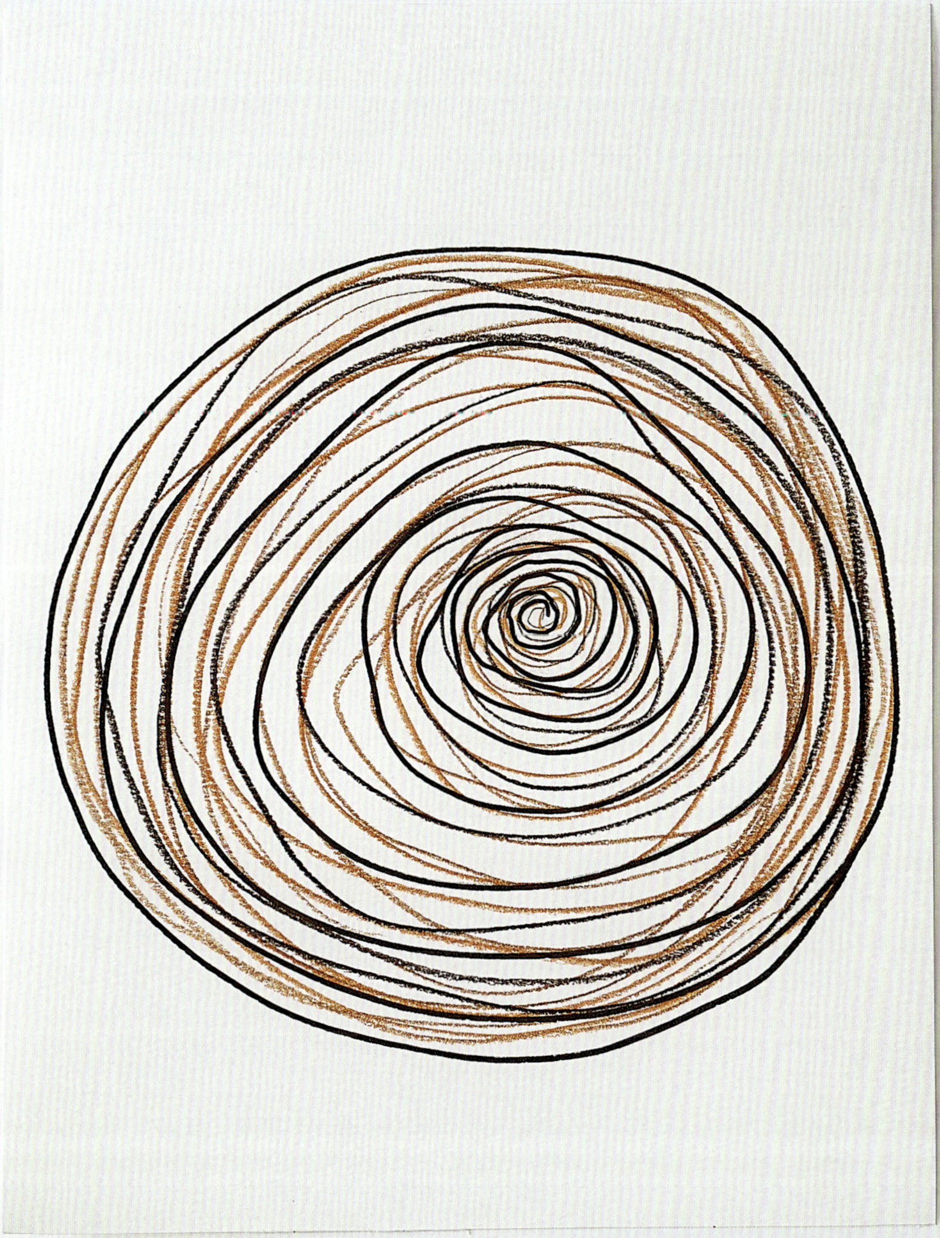

EXERCISE 52

Affirmation poster

Creating visual affirmations reinforces positive beliefs. It engages both creativity and repetition, helping your brain rewire and move towards self-trust and optimism.

INSTRUCTIONS

1. Write one or more positive statements that speak to you – for example 'I am worthy of calm.'
2. Decorate the page around the statements with colours, lines or shapes that feel empowering.
3. Keep it simple, bold and personal.
4. When you finish, display the result.
5. Read your affirmation poster each morning to give you encouragement.

WHAT YOU NEED

⇛ Paper or card

⇛ Markers or paint and brush

THERAPIST'S INSIGHT

By focusing on positive thoughts with affirming statements, the brain rewires itself over time to become predisposed towards positive thoughts. This, in turn, influences your emotional and behavioural responses.

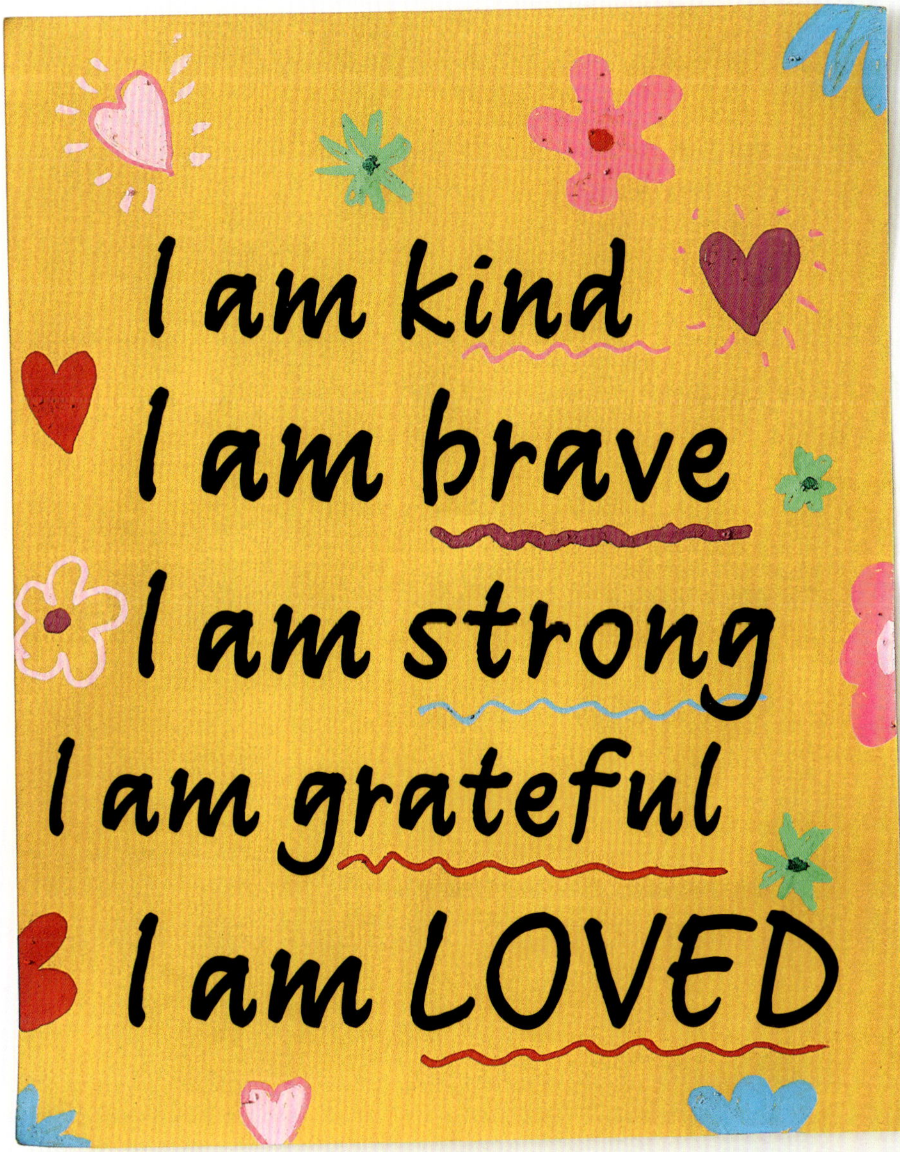
I am kind
I am brave
I am strong
I am grateful
I am LOVED

EXERCISE 53

Celebration confetti

Celebrating small wins boosts dopamine and confidence. It reminds you that joy does not need to wait for big milestones – it is in the everyday moments.

INSTRUCTIONS

1. In a notepad, write down small moments that you are proud of – things you have achieved or have simply survived. Set the notepad aside.
2. Using coloured paper or tissue paper, assign each thing you are proud of a colour. Cut or tear the paper into pieces in any shape you like.
3. Glue these pieces of 'confetti' randomly onto a piece of paper.
4. Let it feel playful and light.
5. Keep the final piece nearby to remind you of your progress.

WHAT YOU NEED

- ⇛ Notepad
- ⇛ Paper
- ⇛ Coloured paper or tissue paper
- ⇛ Scissors (optional)
- ⇛ Glue stick

THERAPIST'S INSIGHT

Whether an achievement is big or small, acknowledging it releases dopamine from the reward system in our brains. This hormone enhances our mood, raises our motivation and reinforces positive behaviours.

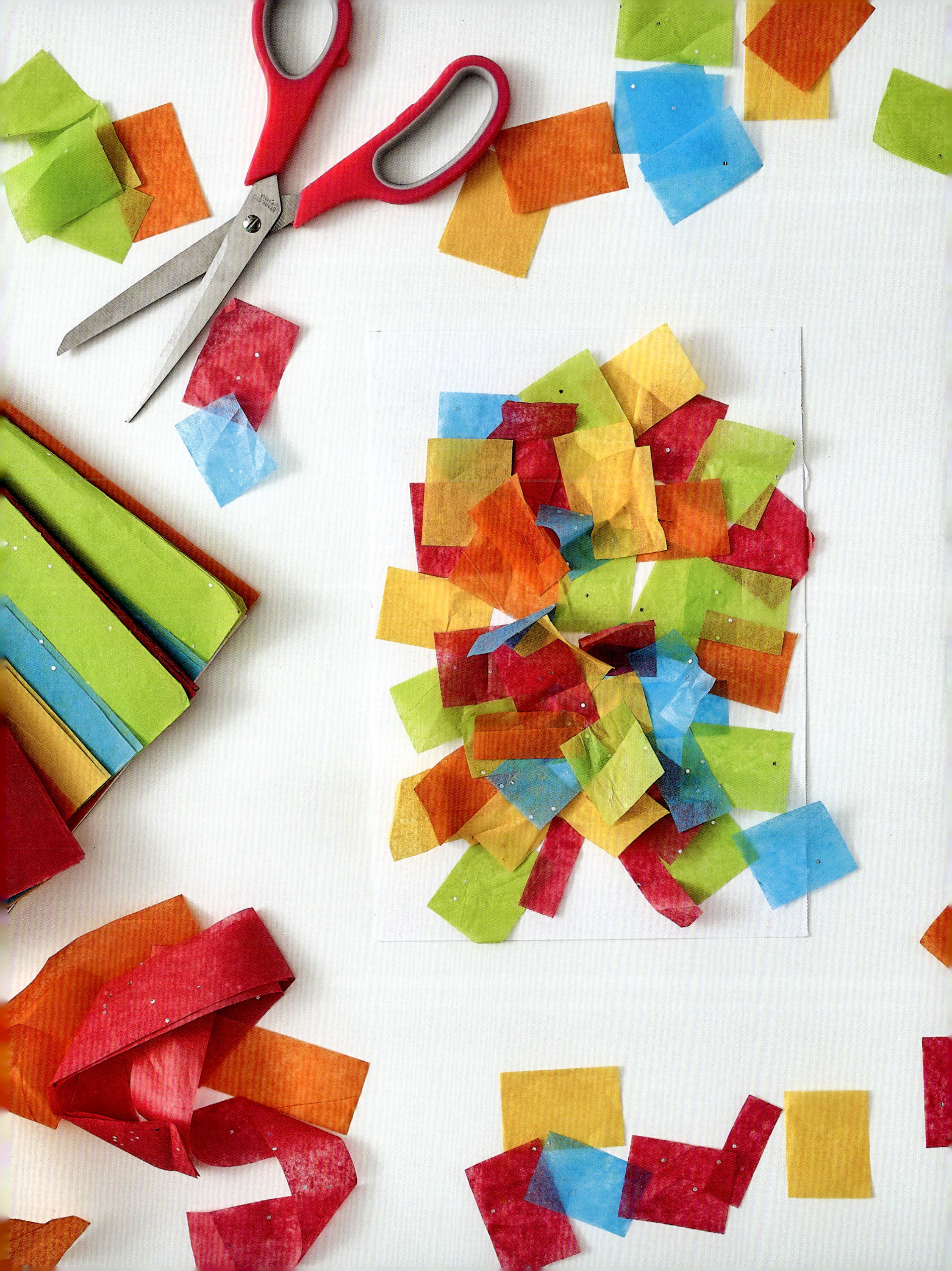

EXERCISE 54

Fruitful study

This exercise strengthens presence and calms an overstimulated mind. Observing a simple object deeply – looking at its textures, shapes and colours – nurtures mindfulness and appreciation for small, quiet beauty.

INSTRUCTIONS

1. Place the fruit in front of you. Spend a few minutes observing its colour, texture and shape. Notice its imperfections.
2. Begin drawing the fruit slowly – curve by curve and shape by shape.
3. Focus on what your eyes actually see, not what you think a fruit looks like.
4. Allow your hand to move at the same gentle pace as your breath.
5. Stop when the act of observing feels complete.

WHAT YOU NEED

- ⇛ Paper
- ⇛ Your favourite art materials – anything you enjoy using
- ⇛ A piece of fruit (such as an apple, pear or orange)
- ⇛ Timer (optional)

THERAPIST'S INSIGHT

Grounding helps bring attention back to the present moment. By focusing carefully on what is in front of you, this exercise can calm racing thoughts, reduce overwhelm and support more balanced thinking.

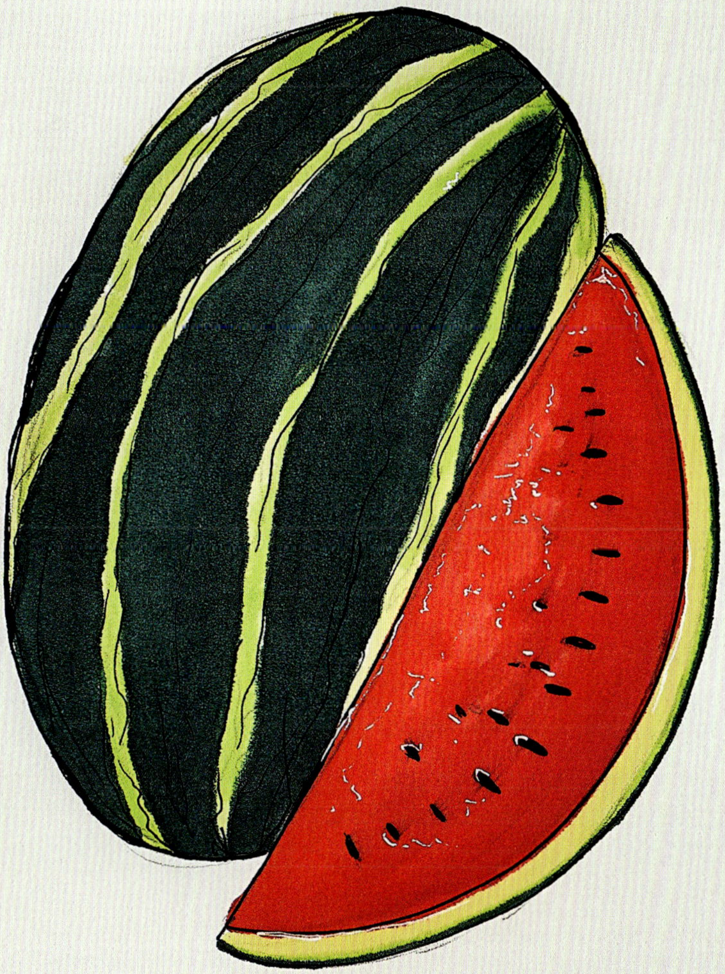

EXERCISE 55

Flowers as feelings

Flowers are powerful mirrors for emotion. Their shapes, colours and fragility reflect our inner world. Translating emotions through organic forms encourages expression, compassion and emotional regulation – helping you see sensitivity as something gentle and beautiful.

INSTRUCTIONS

1. Select a flower that you feel drawn to. Observe its shape, notice where its petals open, overlap or curve, and appreciate how long its stem is.
2. Assign an emotion to this flower – for example, you may feel tenderness, calm or hope.
3. Paint or draw the flower in a way that expresses that feeling. Let the flower and its qualities guide your movements using gentle, flowing lines and soft blending.
4. Stop when the piece feels emotionally complete.

WHAT YOU NEED

⇛ Paper

⇛ Pens or paint and brush

⇛ Fresh flowers or a photo reference

THERAPIST'S INSIGHT

Flowers often represent gentleness, fragility and sensitivity – qualities tied to our more vulnerable self that we may hesitate to share. Looking at a flower invites a softer, more compassionate relationship with our inner self, creating a sense of psychological and emotional safety.

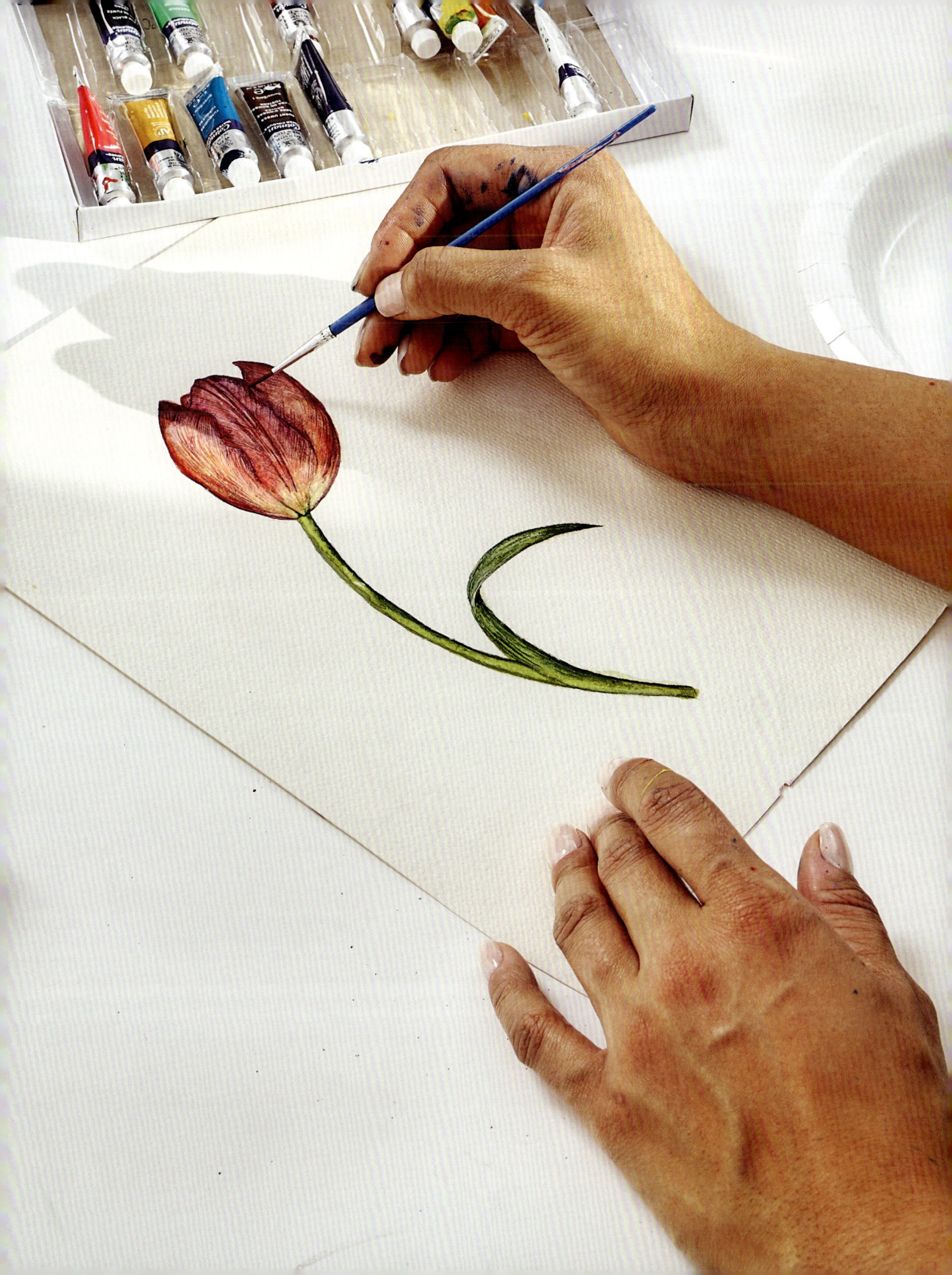

Acknowledgements

I'm so grateful to everyone who helped to bring this book to life. Thank you to the team at Octopus Publishing Group for your belief and guidance, to Jovanna Penney for your insight and support, and to Mark Albini and Elijah Edwards for capturing this work so beautifully. Finally, to my community – thank you for trusting me and for being part of this journey.

Further reading

BOOKS

Magsamen, S and Ross, I, *Your Brain on Art: How the Arts Transform Us*, London: Canongate Books, 2025.

WEBSITES

https://balancedawakening.com/blog/how-art-therapy-fuels-neuroplasticitynbsp (accessed 23 March 2026)

https://drexel.edu/news/archive/2017/june/making-art-activates-brains-reward-pathways (accessed 23 March 2026)

https://www.re-origin.com/articles/somatic-exercises#elementor-toc__heading-anchor-4 (accessed 23 March 2026)

https://my.clevelandclinic.org/health/body/22279-vagus-nerve (accessed 23 March 2026)

https://sleepspace.com/what-are-delta-waves/ (accessed 23 March 2026)

https://traumahealing.org/se-101/ (accessed 23 March 2026)

https://www.cincinnaticenterfordbt.com/coping-with-the-container-method/ (accessed 23 March 2026)

https://www.coswaycbt.co.ukpost/a-metaphor-for-neuroplasticity (accessed 23 March 2026)

https://www.seasonsofgrowthcounseling.com/blog/resourcing-emdr-therapy (accessed 23 March 2026)

https://www.xpandhealth.com/blog/sensory-grounding (accessed 23 March 2026)

JOURNAL ARTICLES

Zhang, X, Wen, K, Ding, H and Zhou, X, 'Experiencing art creation as a therapeutic intervention to relieve anxiety – a case study of a university's ceramic art course', *Frontiers in Psychiatry*, https://pmc.ncbi.nlm.nih.gov/articles/PMC10954310/, 15:1334240, 4 March 2024 (accessed 23 March 2026)

Uvnäs-Moberg, K, Handlin, L and Petersson, M, 'Self-soothing behaviors with particular reference to oxytocin release induced by non-noxious sensory stimulation', *Frontiers in Psychology*, https://pmc.ncbi.nlm.nih.gov/articles/PMC4290532/, 5:1529, 12 January 2015 (accessed 23 March 2026)

Choi, H, Hahm, S-C, Jeon, Y-H, Han, J-W, Kim, S-Y and Woo, J-M, 'The effects of mindfulness-based mandala coloring, made in nature, on chronic widespread musculoskeletal pain: Randomized trial', *Healthcare*, https://pmc.ncbi.nlm.nih.gov/articles/PMC8226655/, 9(6):642, 28 May 2021 (accessed 23 March 2026)

Patrick, D J, 'Somatic experiencing and expressive arts therapy to support autonomic regulation in trauma treatment with adults: a literature review', *Expressive Therapies Capstone Theses*, https://digitalcommons.lesley.edu/expressive_theses/418, 418, 22 May 2021 (accessed 23 March 2026)

Jung, Y and Walther, D B, 'Neural representations in the prefrontal cortex are task dependent for scene attributes but not for scene categories', *The Journal of Neuroscience*, https://www.jneurosci.org/content/41/34/7234, 41 (34) 7234–7245, 25 August 2021 (accessed 23 March 2026)